RECENT ADVANCES IN THE FIELD OF VENTRICULAR ASSIST DEVICES

Edited by **Kazuo Komamura**

Recent Advances in the Field of Ventricular Assist Devices

http://dx.doi.org/10.5772/46016
Edited by Kazuo Komamura

Contributors

Rachit Shah, Megha Goyal, Suchi Shah, Rohit Arora, Anit Mankad, Sharath Kommu, Geetha Bhat, Ashim Aggarwal, Mukesh Gopalakrishnan, Kazuo Komamura, Myra Coppage, Sabino Scolletta, Bonizella Biagioli, Federico Franchi, Luigi Muzzi

Published by InTech

Janeza Trdine 9, 51000 Rijeka, Croatia

Publishing Process Manager Sandra Bakic
Typesetting InTech DTP Team
Cover InTech Design Team

Additional hard copies can be obtained from orders@intechopen.com

Recent Advances in the Field of Ventricular Assist Devices, Edited by Kazuo Komamura
p. cm.
ISBN 978-953-51-1111-5

For EU product safety concerns:
IN TECH d.o.o., Prolaz Marije Krucifikse Kozulić 3, 51000 Rijeka, Croatia,
info@intechopen.com or visit our website at intechopen.com.

Meet the editor

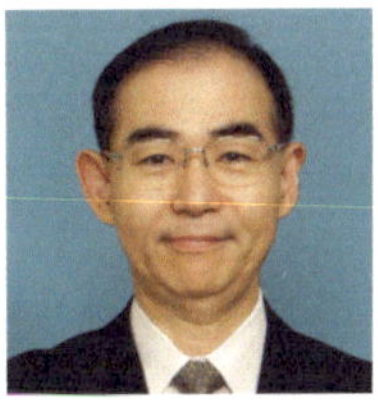

Professor Kazuo Komamura received his medical degree from Osaka University School of Medicine, Japan in 1983. He was trained in Coronary Care Unit, Osaka Police Hospital, Japan. Then, he went abroad to study cellular and molecular mechanisms of heart failure at Prof. Stephen Vatner's Laboratory in Cardiovascular Medicine, Harvard Medical School, U.S.A. Coming back to Japan, he was promoted to the Head, Laboratory of Cardiac Dynamics, National Cerebral and Cardiovascular Centre. In 2008, he became a Professor of Pharmaceutical Sciences, Hyogo University of Health Sciences. Currently, he is working as the Director of Osaka Infirmary, Takeda Pharmaceutical, Company Limited as well as an Adjunct Assistant Professor, Cardiovascular Division, Hyogo College of Medicine, Japan. His research focus is on the development of novel therapies for refractory heart failure. He is now a Fellow of the American College of Cardiology, American Heart Association, European Society of Cardiology and American College of Physicians.

Contents

Preface

Recent developments in ventricular assist devices have been quite remarkable. Rapid advances have been made particularly in terms of smaller size and more durable material and design. As a result, ventricular assist devices are increasingly being implanted in children and they are increasingly being used as a means of destination therapy for elderly patients with heart failure who are not eligible for heart transplantation. New issues have arisen as a result of these expanded indications. This book focuses on recent advances in ventricular assist devices itself and related issues.

The book is divided into two sections. In Section 1, Dr. Rachit Shah and his colleagues describe recent technical advances in ventricular assist devices as well as current indications, their clinical outcomes and countermeasures against complications. Dr. Sabino Scolletta and his colleagues describe the latest techniques to identify the mechanical performance and clinical effectiveness as well as complications of ventricular assist devices at the patient's bedside in real time basis.

Bleeding seems to be an unavoidable complication of ventricular assist devices. Gastrointestinal bleeding in particular is considered to be inevitable in usage of a continuous flow pump. In Section 2, Dr. Geetha Bhat and colleagues describe the current status of and countermeasures against gastrointestinal bleeding along with options for the future research. Allosensitization can result from high-speed rotation of continuous flow pump as well as blood transfusion. Dr. Myra Coppage describes the current state of research on allosensitization including her own, and options for future research. Unlike other chapters, Dr. Kazuo Komamura and his colleagues do not discuss ventricular assist device itself. They describe preliminary results of concurrent use of a new adjunct therapy in combination with ventricular assist devices, and also suggest options for the future research.

The editor hopes that this book will provide valuable and up-to-date information on research and clinical use of ventricular assist devices, and will enable readers to comprehend this fast-growing and exciting field.

Kazuo Komamura, MD, PhD, FACC, FAHA, FESC, FACP
Adjunct Assistant Professor, Cardiovascular Division,
Department of Internal Medicine, Hyogo College of Medicine,
Nishinomiya, Japan

Section 1

Development and Monitoring of the Performance of Ventricular Assist Devices

Chapter 1

Ventricular Assist Devices: Expanding Role for Long Term Cardiac Support

Rachit M. Shah, Megha Goyal, Suchi Shah,
Sharath Kommu, Anit Mankad and Rohit R. Arora

Additional information is available at the end of the chapter

http://dx.doi.org/10.5772/55822

1. Introduction

There are more than 5 million people in United States who are diagnosed with heart failure and about 670,000 new cases occur every year in person age > 45 yrs [1]. HF incidence approaches to 10 per 1,000 of population after the age of 65 yrs. It is the most common hospital discharge diagnosis for patients in this age group [1,2]. There have been a number of significant advances in the treatment of heart failure particularly in pharmacological therapy, but despite that many patients become refractory to medical therapy and develop end stage heart failure. About 50,000- 100,000 patients develop end stage heart failure annually and their prognosis remains poor. [1, 2] When HF is refractory to medical therapy than in appropriate candidates, cardiac transplantation is the most effective treatment modality with average survival of 85% at one year. However, the supply of donor hearts is limited. There is also an increase in the number of heart failure patients who are not candidates for cardiac transplantation, mainly due to older age and presence of co-morbidities. [3,4] This has lead to a considerable interest in alternative forms of cardiac replacement therapy like total artificial hearts and ventricular assist devices. In the last few years, ventricular assist devices (VADs) have emerged as an important therapeutic options for patients with advanced heart Failure. The main purpose of a VAD is to unload the failing heart and help maintain forward cardiac output and vital organ perfusion. Originally introduced as a bridge to recovery, and then as bridge to transplantation, VADs have now evolved into permanent or destination therapy for a growing no. of patients with refractory heart failure. [3-5].

2. History and progress in the field of VADs

The first successful cardiac-assist device in humans was implanted by DeBakey at the Texas Heart Institute in 1966 [5]. Early devices were large and cumbersome with extracorporeal placement and provided temporary support only. The technological advancements led to the development of pulsatile LVAD design pioneered in 1976 as the Axio-symmetrical and Pierce-Donachy LVADs. A refined version of the latter device known as the Heartmate (Thoratec) was approved by the FDA as a bridging device to cardiac transplantation in 1994 [5]. Its updated version, the Heartmate XVE was approved as bridge therapy in 1998. The Randomized Evaluation of Mechanical Assistance in Treatment of Chronic Heart Failure (REMATCH) study evaluated the long term benefit of Heartmate XVE placement compared with optimal medical therapy in end-stage heart failure patients.(4) There was 48% reduction in death from all causes, attributable to LVAD therapy compared with best medical therapy in this trial. On this basis, the Heartmate XVE was approved for use as destination therapy in 2002. With time VADs have evolved significantly, with three major changes to date: (*a*) Transition from pulsatile to continuous-flow devices; (*b*) Reduction in size with the preference for internal placement of the devices; (*c*) Use of electricity as a power source [6].The newest continuous-flow VADs are much smaller in size and owing to less moving parts are silent in operation, leading to significantly greater patient satisfaction and making this therapy more favorable for long-term support. Many newer VADs have been approved by FDA in recent years which includes but not limited to Thoratec Heartmate II (approved in Jan,2010), Heartware Venricular assist System (approved in Nov,2012) and Jarvic 2000 (approved in Aug,2012).

3. Overview of VADs

3.1. Components of a VAD

VADs support the failing heart by unloading the ventricle and generating flow to the systemic and/or pulmonary circulation. They can be used to support the left ventricle, right ventricle or both the ventricles. LVAD is the main assist device used in clinical practice. Use of isolated right ventricular assist device (RVAD) is a rare event [7]. It is usually inserted around the time of placement of a left ventricular assist device (LVAD) to provide biventricular assistance. Unlike a single VAD, biventricular mechanical devices create a complex system with 2 independent pumps, one right sided and the other left sided which supports both left and right ventricles.

VAD typically has an inflow cannula, an outflow cannula, a pumping chamber, per-cutaneous driveline, a controller and power supply [7]. VADs are usually implanted through a median sternotomy. The inflow cannula is connected to the heart and it decompresses the ventricular cavity and an outflow cannula returns blood to either the ascending aorta or the main pulmonary artery. (9). The pumping chamber of the VAD is implanted sub-diaphragmatically to a pre-peritoneal or intra-abdominal position or may be situated in a para-corporeal position outside the body [7]. A percutaneous driveline, containing the control and power wires, is tunneled through the skin of the abdominal wall. It connects the device to an external portable driver consisting of an electronic or pneumatic controller and a power supply that may be worn around the waist, carried in a shoulder bag, or contained within a small bedside monitor [7].

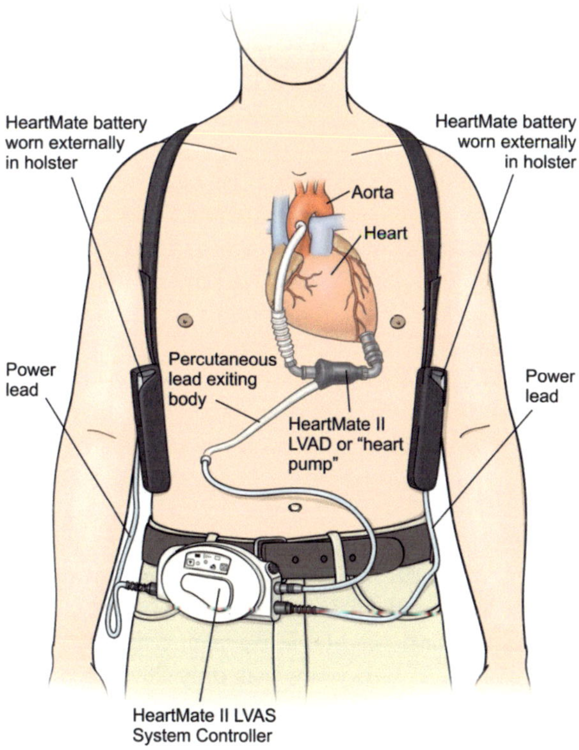

Figure 1. Image showing various components of a Heart Mate II ventricular assist device: Inflow and outflow canula, Heartmate II pump, percutaneous driveline, External portable driver (System controller) (Photo courtesy Thoratec).

3.2. Types of VADs

Many VADs are currently available commercially or in various stages of development. These are developed to satisfy special needs for either short or longer-term support and, therefore, differ markedly in their design characteristics, principles of operation, hemodynamic capabilities, method of insertion, and durability.

3.2.1. Percutaneous short term devices

Percutaneous VADs include devices that are inserted through the femoral artery and advanced to the left ventricle. Examples include Impella 2.5 pump and TandemHeart. Impella 2.5 pump (Abiomed Inc., Danvers, MA) is an Impeller-driven, axial flow pump, capable of pumping 2.5 L/min [8,9]. TandemHeart (CardiacAssist, Inc., Pittsburgh, PA) is a low speed centrifugal continuous-flow pump that drains oxygenated blood through a catheter advanced across the interatrial septum to the left atrium and pumps it back to one or both femoral arteries [10,11].

3.2.2. Longer term assist devices

The currently available longer-term VADs are categorized into three generations, reflecting the order in which they were developed and the type of pumping mechanism they use.

3.2.2.1. First generation or pulsatile flow pumps

These are pulsatile devices that use pusher plates and have inflow and outflow valves. These devices are efficacious at unloading the left ventricle and maintaining the circulation, with the capacity to pump up to 10 L/min [6]. Examples include the HeartMate® I or XVE (Thoratec Corp., Pleasanton, CA) and the Novacor VAD (WorldHeart Inc., Oakland, California, USA). These implantable VADs are placed intra-abdominally or pre-peritoneally in a pocket under the abdominal rectus muscle and connected to the apex of the left ventricle and to the ascending aorta [12]. There is increased risk of hematomas and infections as they are large in volume, requiring extensive surgical dissection. The percutaneous leads of these devices, especially those of the HeartMate XVE, are large and stiff and contain an air vent channel, which makes the system quite noisy and uncomfortable [12]. All pulsatile devices have biological or mechanical valves to allow a unidirectional blood flow. Anticoagulation is necessary for all devices, except the HeartMate XVE due to a textured inner surface of the pump stimulating formation of a biological layer preventing thrombus formation [11]. After the REMATCH study, Heartmate XVE was approved for use as "destination therapy" in 2002. Although the VAD therapy group had significantly greater survival and quality of life at both one and two years of follow-up, the survival at two years was only 28%. In addition, there were large numbers of readmissions and device-related complications including sepsis and stroke. Therefore, use of Heartmate XVE as destination has not been widely accepted [11]. The first generation devices are also used successfully as a "bridge to transplantation" with a perio-perative mortality of 15–20% and an overall survival until device explantation of 60–70%. However, in the majority of studies, the maximal support duration does not exceed 6 months, and in most studies mean support duration ranges only from 50 to 60 days [13-15]. Survival and quality of life has been closely related to adverse events such as bleeding, infections, thrombo-embolic events and technical failures.

3.2.2.2. Second generation or continuous (axial) flow pumps

The second generation VADs are much smaller and durable in comparison to the first generation devices. The examples iclude the HeartMate 2 VAD (Thoratec Inc.), the Jarvik 2000 (Jarvik Heart Inc., New York, New York), Micromed Debakey VAD and the Berlin Heart Incor (Berlin Heart AG) [11]. They have the continuous flow impeller pumps which are considerably smaller and safer to insert. Because they have only one moving part (the rotor), they are expected to be more durable than first-generation devices. To maintain an international normalized ratio (INR) of 2.0–2.5, the use of these pumps requires full anticoagulant therapy coupled with antiplatelet medications, such as aspirin or clopidogrel [11]. The HeartMate 2 is the most successful second-generation device with over 2500 implants worldwide. It is one-

http://dx.doi.org/10.5772/55822

seventh of the size and one-fourth the weight of the HeartMate XVE. Heartmate II device has been approved by the US FDA for implantation as BTT in April 2008 and as DT in January 2010 [11,12]. The mean duration of support reported from the use of these continuous flow, rotary pumps is considerably longer compared with the first-generation devices (166–236 vs. 50–60 days). Studies show 2 years survival of 65 and 69% with no mechanical failure and low fatal adverse event rates. The incidence of thrombo-embolic events in HeartMate 2 patients is in most studies comparable with those seen with Heart- Mate XVE, however the risk of hemorrhagic stroke rates tend to be higher (2–3%), as a result of the anticoagulation [12].

3.2.2.3. Third generation or continuous (centrifugal) flow pumps

Third-generation VADs are small centrifugal pumps in which the rotor is magnetically or mechanically suspended and, therefore, does not use ball bearings. Drivelines are less thick and more flexible. These features, coupled with the lower number of revolutions per minute, should enhance durability in comparison with the second generation pumps. Examples of such third generation VADs are the VentrAssist VAD (Ventracor Ltd, Chatswood, New South Wales, Australia) [16] and the DuraHeart (Terumo, Somerset, New Jersey, USA) [17]. These devices are thought to last as long as 5–10 years, and their performance is being evaluated in several phase I studies involving the HVAD® (Heart- Ware, Miramar, FL) devices, and more recently the DuraHeart® (Terumo Kabushiki Kaisha, Tokyo, Japan) system. They still carry the risk of neurological complications like stroke as well as risk of infections [11,12].

3.3. Indications for VADs

VADs can be used for a wide spectrum of diseases based on the therapeutic goals of circulatory support as well as the duration of treatment. The major three indications include:

1. Bridge to recovery
2. Bridge to transplantation
3. Destination therapy

4. Bridge to recovery

As name suggests it implies the use of VADs in patients who need only temporary support to provide mechanical unloading of the heart as in cases of acute cardiogenic or post-cardiotomy shock, acute inflammatory cardiomyopathies, and myocardial infarction. This will allow sufficient time for myocardial recovery and eventual removal of device. The ability of LVADs to support an acutely failing heart while it recovers function, is well documented [16-18]. The VAD causes mechanical unloading of the left ventricle, which leads to a reduction in ventricular size and volumes [19] as well as normalization of pressure-volume relationship curves [20]. It also affects myocardial structure by altering both cellular and extracellular component which contributes to recovery of myocardial function at cellular level [21-24]. This process of recovery of ventricular structure and function with the use of VADs is known as 'Reverse remodeling'.

5. Molecular pathways for reverse remodeling

VAD therapy has shown to affect excitation contraction (E-C) coupling in myocardial cells [25]. After VAD treatment, cardiomyocyte contractility is increased [26,27] and the force-frequency relationship is normalized [28,29]. Action-potential duration is also reduced [30,31] mirroring the shortening of the QT interval on electrocardiogram [32]. In addition to E-C coupling mechanisms, several other molecular mechanisms responsible for VAD-induced reverse remodeling have been described. These include effects at the levels of metabolic pathways, alterations in calcium handling proteins, immune and inflammatory responses, transcription factors, the adrenergic system, cytoskeletal proteins, the extracellular matrix, neurohormonal activation, and apoptosis and necrosis signaling [6]. Clinically these changes improve left ventricular function and patients have a dramatic increase in their exercise capacity following LVAD implantation. These findings encouraged the explantation of LVADs in select patients who have demonstrated sufficient recovery of myocardial function. To date clinical results are mixed and although the large number of studies report regression or normalization of the pathological substrate following VAD treatment, the clinical evidence for recovery remains limited. To date, an average of only 5%–10% of patients who undergo mechanical circulatory support demonstrate adequate recovery of ventricular function to allow device explantation [6].

There is also concern that prolonged mechanical unloading reduces cardiac cell function, as well as cell size, in a time-dependent manner which may lead to myocardial atrophy [20-24]. Unloading induced atrophy can be an important impediment to myocardial recovery and removal of the VADs for bridge-to-recovery, limiting the efficacy of VAD treatment [33]. Minimizing unloading-induced atrophy may be an important strategy to obtain the beneficial effects of VADs and, to this end, a pharmacological regimen that includes clenbuterol has been tested in combination with VAD treatment [34-36]. Clenbuterol is a β2 adrenoceptor agonist that is currently approved only for patients with asthma, but has been shown in animal models to induce hypertrophy of skeletal and cardiac muscle and enhanced mechanical strength of contraction. In a study, a novel combination regimen which included clenbuterol was used in patients with non-ischemic cardiomyopathy who were transplant candidates and required a VAD for refractory heart failure [34-36]. In nearly 70% of patients on the combination therapy, the VAD could be removed within one year. After four years of follow-up, the average ejection fraction had improved from 15% preoperatively to 62%. These encouraging data have prompted the initiation of the Harefield Recovery Protocol Study (HARPS) to assess clinical cardiac recovery and explore molecular mechanisms of clenbuterol [6].

6. Bridge to transplantation

"Bridge-to-transplantation" is the strategy in which VADs are used for improving ventricular function and peripheral perfusion in patients awaiting cardiac transplantation. Several studies have demonstrated that VADs ensure sustained improvement in hemodynamic status and quality of life in patients awaiting cardiac transplantation [37]. More than 80% of VAD-treated patients undergoing cardiac transplantation have a normal or improved post-transplant outcome [38].

When implanted in patients refractory to medical therapy, LVADs lead to improved end organ function as well as overall physical conditioning [11]. LVAD markedly decreases the filling pressures and increases cardiac output by taking over the work of the left ventricle, the. This leads to lower pulmonary vascular resistance and a reduction in afterload for the right ventricle. Additionally, the increase in cardiac output provides additional preload for the right ventricle, which further enhances its function. This improvement in right ventricular function and mechanical replacement of left ventricular output by LVAD results in more efficient delivery of oxygen to end-organ tissues. As a result, the presence of the LVAD can partially or totally reverse functional impairment of these organs. This is most clearly evident in the kidneys, in which renal failure can improve or resolve following the implantation of an LVAD. All organ systems benefit from the increase in perfusion, allowing sick patients to stabilize or improve as they wait for a heart transplant. In addition to providing an increased length of time on the organ waiting list, LVADs significantly improve outcomes by reducing patients' co morbidities at the time of transplant. This makes them better transplant candidates and improves their post transplant outcomes [11, 12].

7. Destination therapy

In "Destination Therapy",VADs are used as an alternative to cardiac transplant to support the patients for their entire life. It involves the largest population of the patients with end stage heart failure who are unable to receive cardiac transplantation [39]. The success of LVAD implantation as "Bridge to transplantation" (BTT) in candidates with refractory heart failure led to the investigations for its use as an alternative to Heart transplantation. The REMATCH trial was one of the most remarkable trials that assessed the feasibility of VADs for Destination Therapy (DT) [40]. The trial was conducted between May 1998 and July 2001 at 20 US hospitals and it *showed significant improvement of the quality of life in patients supported with LVAD and improved one year survival from 25% to 52%. These data led to the US Food and Drug Administration (FDA) approval of the modified HeartMate XVE LVAD for use as DT in November 2002, thus launching a new era of surgical therapy for advanced heart failure* [39,40*].* One of the more recent trials, the Heartmate II trial was conducted between March 2005 and May 2007 and it has shown that patients supported with HM II VAD (continuous flow VAD) had significantly improved two-year survival when compared to HM XVE recipients (58% vs. 24%, respectively) and significantly improved probability of freedom from stroke and device failure at two years, as compared to the recipients of pulsatile devices. These data led to approval of Heartmate II VAD for DT by US FDA in January 2010 [39,40].

8. Indications for DT

The criteria for VAD implantation for DT are based largely on the entry criteria into the REMATCH trial [40]. They are:

1. Class IV NYHA symptoms for at least 60 of the last 90 days despite maximized oral therapy, including dietary salt restriction, diuretics, digitalis, beta-blockers, and angiotensin converting enzyme (ACE) inhibitors (if tolerated), or requirement of inotropic support as outlined by the AHA/ACC guidelines for heart failure treatment.
2. LVEF of ≤25%,
3. Peak oxygen consumption of <12 mL/kg/min or documented inability to wean intravenous inotropic therapy owing to symptomatic hypotension, decreasing renal function, or worsening pulmonary congestion.
4. Contraindication to HT due to either age greater than 65 years or comorbidities such as insulin-dependent diabetes mellitus with end-organ damage, chronic renal failure, or others, and
5. Appropriate body size (≥1.5 m2) to support the LVAD implantation.

9. Survival with DT

As mentioned earlier the results of the REMATCH trial revealed significant improvement in one-year survival from 25% to 52%.with improvement of the quality of life in patients supported with VAD in comparison with optical medical therapy. In the post rematch era despite improvements in design, there was no significant improvement in clinical outcomes with pulsatile flow devices [39]. Recently published Heart Mate II trial showed that patients supported with continuous flow HM II LVAD had significantly improved two-year survival when compared to pulsatile flow HM XVE recipients (58% vs. 24%, respectively) and significantly improved probability of freedom from stroke and device failure at two years, as compared to the recipients of pulsatile devices[40].

Experiences of the post-REMATCH era have shown that many DT recipients who were initially deemed not transplantable have improved their condition and became eligible for HT; 1 in every 5 recipients of HM XVE in the post-REMATCH era (17% of the 280 studied patients) underwent successful HT within 10 months from device implant [6]. In most of these cases the improvements occurred due to the resolution of deemed irreversible pulmonary hypertension, recovery of renal function, weight loss, achieving cancer-free period, or reversal of other conditions. Therefore, one should not assume that DT would in the future preclude transplantation [39]. Although LVAD implantation in the post-REMATCH era continues to be associated with substantial survival benefit as compared to medical therapy, the outcomes of DT remain substantially inferior to those of HT (85% one-year survival) [39].

Contraindications for LVAD [41,42] therapy

- Irreversible contraindication for heart transplantation if recovery or destination is not the aim
- Biventricular failure in patients older than 65 years
- High surgical risk for successful implantation

- Recent or evolving stroke
- Neurological deficits impairing the ability to manage device
- Significant underlying psychiatric illness or lack of social support that may impair ability to maintain and operate VAD
- Active systemic infection or major chronic risk for infection
- Fixed pulmonary or portal hypertension
- Severe pulmonary dysfunction (eg, FEV_1 <1 L)
- Impending renal or hepatic failure
- Multisystem organ failure
- Inability to tolerate anticoagulation
- Heparin-induced thrombocytopenia

Relative contraindications

- Age >65 years, unless minimal or no other clinical risk factors
- Morbid obesity (BMI>40 kg/m2)
- Chronic kidney disease with serum creatinine level >3.0 mg/dL
- Severe mitral stenosis or moderate to severe aortic insufficiency, or uncorrectable mitral regurgitation
- Severe chronic malnutrition (BMI <21 kg/m2 in males and <19 kg/m2 in females)

10. Complications associated with VAD therapy

VAD therapy is associated with various long term complications which include bleeding (epistaxis or GI bleed), pump thrombosis, right sided heart failure, arrhythmias, hemolytic anemia etc. It is also associated with perioperative bleeding and infections as well as complications like air embolism and sepsis. The major late complications are mechanical device failure, neurologic events, and infections [43,11].

1. Mechanical Failure:

Device malfunction is an important cause of morbidity and mortality in patients living with VADs, especially with the prolonged support required for both bridge to transplantation and destination therapy [44-46]. In the REMATCH trial, 35% of patients experienced component failure within 24 months of implantation [11]. A contemporary review of 109 pulsatile VADs implanted at a single institution found that the probability of device failure was 6%, 12%, 27%, and 64% at 6 months, 1 year, 18 months, and 2 years, respectively [11]. On the other hand for continuous flow pumps the mechanical durability seems to be markedly improved. In one study on patients with a HeartMate II VAD as bridge to transplantation, only 5 of 133 (4%) developed either device thrombosis or a complication from surgical implantation necessitating device replacement.

Complications can arise in any component from the portable drive/system controller that controls and powers the device to the inflow and outflow cannulae, valves and batteries [11]. These devices have system controllers and monitors that provide visual and auditory alarms during malfunction. To diagnose suspected device malfunction these alarms must be used in conjunction with clinical, laboratory, and imaging data. For troubleshooting, various catheter, angiography, fluoroscopy, and echocardiography based protocols have been developed to help diagnose common malfunctions [45,46]. If necessary, repair of a dysfunctional VAD or removal and replacement with a new VAD may be performed.

Role of echocardiography in detecting VAD related complications

Echocardiography is one of the important diagnostic tools in detecting VAD related complications. On many instances, it is used as the test of choice in outpatient setting to detect the complications as well as to adjust VAD parameters. Following are some of the examples of complications which can be detected by echocardiography [45,46,59].

- RV failure (decreased RV systolic function, increased RV size, increased right atrial pressure, and increased tricuspid regurgitation)
- Pericardial effusion with or without cardiac tamponade
- LVAD-related continuous aortic insufficiency (aortic regurgitation throughout cardiac diastole and systole)
- Inadequate LV filling (small LV dimensions)
- LVAD-induced ventricular tachycardia (underfilled LV and mechanical impact with septum)
- Intracardiac thrombus (including right and left atrial, LV apical, and aortic root thrombus)
- Continuous pump apical inflow abnormality due to inflow cannula obstruction, malposition, or hyperdynamic apical LV function (color Doppler high-velocity aliased flow at the cannula orifice with a peak Doppler velocity >2 m/s)
- Pulsatile pump apical inflow obstruction (intermittent interruption of usual laminar LVAD diastolic inflow using pulsed-wave Doppler with inflow velocities >2.5 m/s and color flow aliasing at the cannula orifice)
- Pulsatile pump inflow valve regurgitation (apical inflow cannula turbulent flow detected by color Doppler during LVAD ejection, dilated LV,frequent opening of the AV, and reduced outflow graft flow <1.8 m/s)
- Cannula kinking or complete thrombosis (loss of Doppler signal in all echo views and loss of RV outflow tract stroke volume with speed change)

- Hypertensive emergency, continuous flow pump (minimal AV opening, dilated LV, worsening MR, and peak outflow cannula velocity >2 m/s)
- Impeller cessation, continuous flow pump (dilated LV, acute reversal of apical inflow flow direction using spectral or color Doppler, worsening MR, and decreased RV outflow tract stroke volume).

2. Neurologic Events:

Neurologic complications from VAD therapy include cerebro-vascular accidents (both ischemic infarcts and intracranial hemorrhage) as well as non stroke complications like syncope, seizure, brain abscesses, and encephalopathy. Implanted mechanical devices are susceptible to thrombo-embolic events due to their unique properties. The foreign surfaces of VADs and associated turbulent flow can activate the immune system, platelets, and the coagulation cascade which increases the risk of thrombi formation [47]. Moreover, unmasking or inadequate treatment of hypertension, older age, higher VAD flow and pulsatility index, and inadequate anticoagulation further increase the risk for development of neurological events. The incidence of CVAs range from 0.009 to 5.73 events per patient-year [47-49]. The prevalence of neurologic events with destination therapy has ranged from 44% in the RE-MATCH trial (HeartMate XVE) to 57% in the European LionHeart Clinical Utility Baseline Study [11].

Not all devices have the same neurologic event rate. Design modifications like the use of novel biologic materials, textured coatings, and a single moving part, are believed to reduce the risk of thrombus formation. Promising data from the HeartMate II trial demonstrated reduced adverse events per patient year with respect to stroke (0.19 vs. 0.44) and non-stroke (0.26 vs. 0.67) neurologic events compared with a pulsatile flow pump [11]. Appropriate device selection, prevention of infection that can activate platelets, blood pressure control, and meticulous regulation of anticoagulation are all critical for the prevention of cerebro-vascular accidents after VAD implantation [50,51].

3. Infections:

VAD infections occur most frequently between 2 weeks and 2 months after implantation. The predominant organisms are Gram-positive organisms *Staphylococcus epidermidis* and *Staphylococcus aureus* followed by enterococci. Other commonly implicated organisms include Gram negative bacilli such as *Pseudomonas aeruginosa, Enterobacter,* and *Klebsiella* species, along with fungi. Frequent use of broad-spectrum antibiotics, particularly during the index hospitalization, is believed to increase susceptibility for fungal infections, which are associated with the highest risk of death [52-58].

The most common site of infection is the percutaneous driveline, which can often be managed successfully with wound care and antibiotics. However, a driveline infection can spread to other components of the VAD resulting in bacteremia, sepsis, and endocarditis. Sepsis in patients with mechanical assist devices has been reported to be the leading cause of death and can result in cerebral emboli and multi-organ failure [52-58]. Other infections, including mediastinitis and peritonitis, have also been reported.

Many strategies have been adopted to try to minimize device-related and wound infections. Proper care of the driveline exit site must be maintained. Strict aseptic technique (e.g., sterile gloves, mask) must be followed when caring for the percutaneous exit site. The site should be gently cleaned with a mild antimicrobial soap and rinsed with sterile normal saline after which a dry sterile dressing should be applied. At all times, the driveline must be secured to minimize the risk of trauma; immobilization can be performed with an abdominal binder, additional gauze, tape, or a stoma-adhesive device [11]. There are also many modifications made to device design to further decrease the risk of infection which include the use of larger single-lead drivelines and drivelines coated with chlorhexidine and silver sulfadiazine. Studies of rotary blood pumps with their reduced surface area for colonization and smaller surgical pump pocket suggest that they are less prone to infection [52-58].

11. Preparing the patients for life outside hospital after VAD implantation

Adequate cardiac rehabilitation including physical, occupational, and nutritional therapy is very important for patient's recovery from VAD implantation.

a. Physical Exercise

It is very important for patients to continue their physical performance. VAD's ability to unload the ventricle leading to profound ventricular pressure and volume changes leads to reversal of neurohormonal activation, impaired metabolic vasodilation, and myocardial remodeling [60].

b. Nutrition

The nutritional status of a VAD patient should be checked periodically. Patients who have malnutrition, particularly cachexia or hypoalbuminemia, may be predisposed to immune system dysfunction, impaired healing, and infection [61,62].

c. Routine self-care

It is important to perform periodic cleaning and maintenance of VAD equipment after discharge including changing the dressing at the exit site, inspecting for signs of infection, measuring daily vital signs, examining the connectors and ventilator filter for dirt or debris, and assessing the status of the batteries [7].

d. Harmful environments

Due to the sensitive nature of these machines, patients should avoid extremes of temperature for prolonged periods of time, operating heavy machinery and must not engage in contact sports or strenuous activities.

e. Responsibility of primary care physicians and nurse associations

Primary health care providers play an important role in successful outpatient management and should be properly instructed in the basic management of VADs. Such providers should be aware of the potential for infection and neurologic complications, as well as pump stoppage.

Primary health care providers should also discuss end of life care options specially for patients who are being considered for "Destination therapy". When patients are considering the VAD therapy, a consult to palliative care team can mobilize important services including symptom management as well as psychological and spiritual support for the patients and their families. After device implant, palliative care team can provide essential support to the patients as needed. If a catastrophic complication occurs after the implant (eg debilitating stroke, overwhelming infection) palliative care experts can play a prominent role in patient management (eg comfort measures, pain control and supportive care) and refer them to hospice care.

f. Role of first responders

Local first responders and emergency department personnel should become familiar with the basic physiology, system operation, and components of a VAD [7].

g. Cardiopulmonary resuscitation and cardioversion

Cardioversion or defibrillation is possible with all technologies, as is intubation. When external defibrillation is required, the VAD system controller should be disconnected before delivering the shock to avoid electronic disruption.

12. Conclusion

With collaboration of multidisciplinary teams composed of engineers, scientists, physicians and nurses, VAD technology and applications continues to evolve. This progress has lead to significant improvement in patient care as well as outcomes of patients receiving this therapy. This technology is becoming a safe alternative to heart transplant for rapidly growing patient population with advance end stage heart failure. With technological advancements, VADs are becoming smaller, more efficient and durable, though challenges are still ahead in making them more safer with less adverse effects. With the encouraging results in terms of survival as well as quality of life, VAD therapy is also being considered for patients with less severe heart failure. As patient population considered for VAD therapy continues to grow, more efforts are needed in educating patients and their families as well as medical care providers to effectively manage the challenges associated with these devices.

Abbreviations

VAD - ventricular assist device

LV- Left ventricle

RV- Right ventricle

LVAD- Left ventricular assist device

RVAD- Right ventricular assist device

FDA- Food and drug administration

BTT - Bridge to transplant

DT- Destination therapy

HF- Heart failure

HT - Heart transplant.

HM XVE- Heart Mate XVE

HM II- Heart Mate II

NYHA- New york heart association

LVEF- Left ventricular ejection fraction

BMI- Body mass index

Author details

Rachit M. Shah*, Megha Goyal, Suchi Shah, Sharath Kommu, Anit Mankad and Rohit R. Arora

*Address all correspondence to: dr_rachit@yahoo.com

Department of Cardiology/Internal Medicine, Virginia Commonwealth University/ Chicago Medical School (Rosalind Franklin University), Chicago, USA

References

[1] Lloyd-jones, D, Adams, R, Carnethon, M, et al. Heart disease and stroke statistics, 2009 update. A report from the american heart association statistics committee and stroke statistics subcommittee. *Circulation* (2009). e, 21-181.

[2] Miller, L. W, & Missov, E. D. Epidemiology of heart failure. *Cardiol Clin* (2001). , 19, 547-55.

[3] Park, S. J, Tector, A, Piccioni, W, et al. Left ventricular assist devices as destination therapy: a new look at survival. *J Thorac Cardiovasc Surg* (2005). , 129, 9-17.

[4] Rose, E. A, Gelijns, A. C, Moskowitz, A. J, et al. Long-term mechanical left ventricular assistance for end-stage heart failure. *N Engl J Med* (2001). , 345, 1435-43.

[5] Barry, A, Boilson, M. B, & Mrcpi, M. D. Eugenia Raichlin, MD, Soon J. Park, MD, and Sudhir S. Kushwaha, MD: Device Therapy and Cardiac Transplantation for End-Stage Heart Failure; *Curr Probl Cardiol*, January (2010).

[6] Cesare, M. Terracciano, LeslieW. Miller, and Magdi H. Yacoub: Contemporary Use of Ventricular Assist Devices. *Annu. Rev. Med* (2010).

[7] Sean, R, Wilson, M. D, Michael, M, Givertz, M. D, Garrick, C, Stewart, M. D, Gilbert, H, & Mudge, J. R. MD. Ventricular Assist DevicesThe Challenges of Outpatient Management; *Journal of American College of Cardiology* (2009). , 54(18)

[8] Henriques, J. P, Remmelink, M, Baan, J, et al. (2006). Safety and feasibility of elective high risk percutaneous coronary intervention procedures with left ventricular support of the Impella Recover LP 2.5. *Am. J. Cardiol. 97*, 990-92.

[9] Thiele, H, Lauer, B, Hambrecht, R, et al. (2001). Reversal of cardiogenic shock by percutaneous left atrialto- femoral arterial bypass assistance. *Circulation 104*, 2917-22.

[10] Henriques, J. P, & De Mol, B. A. (2008). New percutaneous mechanical left ventricular support for acute MI: the AMC MACH program. *Nat. Clin. Pract. Cardiovasc. Med. 5*, 62-63.

[11] Shah, R. M, Kommu, S, Bhuriya, R, Arora, R, et al. Ventricular Assist Device: Emerg ing Modality for Long Term Cardiac Support. Book Chapter. Intech, (2012).

[12] Lahpor, J. R. State of the art: implantable ventricular assist devices; *Current Opinion in Organ Transplantation* (2009).

[13] Frazier, O. H, Rose, E. A, Oz, M. C, Dembitsky, W, et al. Multicenter clinical evaluation of the HeartMate vented electric left ventricular assist system in patients awaiting heart transplantation. *J Thoracic Cardiovasc Surg* (2001). , 122, 1186-1195.

[14] Kalya, A. V, Tector, A. J, Crouch, J. D, et al. Comparison of Novacor and HeartMate vented electric left ventricular assist devices in single institution. *J Heart Lung Transplant* (2005). , 24, 1973-1975.

[15] El-Banayosy, A, Arusoglu, L, Kizner, L, et al. Novacor left ventricular assist systems versus HeartMate vented electric left ventricular system as a long mechanical support device in bridging patients: a prospective study. *J Thoracic Cardiovasc Surg* (2000). , 119, 581-587.

[16] Esmore, D, Kaye, D, Spratt, P, et al. A prospective, multicenter trial of the VentrAssist left ventricular assist device for bridge to transplant, safety and efficacy. *J Heart Lung Transplant* (2008). , 27, 579-588.

[17] Morshuis, M, Banayosy, A, Arusoglu, L, et al. European experience of DuraHeart magnetically levitated centrifugal left ventricular assist system. *Eur J Cardiothorac Surg* (2009). , 35, 1020-1028.

[18] Maybaum, S, Mancini, D, Xydas, S, et al. (2007). Cardiac improvement during mechanical circulatory support: a prospective multicenter study of the LVAD Working Group. *Circulation 115*, 2497-505.

[19] Mancini, D. M, Beniaminovitz, A, Levin, H, et al. (1998). Low incidence of myocardial recovery after left ventricular assist device implantation in patients with chronic heart failure. *Circulation 98*, 2383-89.

[20] Ritter, M, Su, Z, Xu, S, et al. (2000). Cardiac unloading alters contractility and calcium homeostasis in ventricular myocytes. *J. Mol. Cell Cardiol. 32*, 577-84.

[21] Kolar, F. MacNaughton C, Papousek F, et al. (1995). Changes in calcium handling in atrophic heterotopically isotransplanted rat hearts. *Basic Res. Cardiol. 90*, 475-81.

[22] Welsh, D. C, Dipla, K, Mcnulty, P. H, et al. (2001). Preserved contractile function despite atrophic remodelling in unloaded rat hearts. *Am. J. Physiol. Heart Circ. Physiol.* 281:H, 1131-36.

[23] Oriyanhan, W, Tsuneyoshi, H, Nishina, T, et al. (2007). Determination of optimal duration of mechanical unloading for failing hearts to achieve bridge to recovery in a rat heterotopic heart transplantation model. *J. Heart Lung Transplant. 26*, 16-23.

[24] Ito, K, Nakayama, M, Hasan, F, et al. (2003). Contractile reserve and calcium regulation are depressed in myocytes from chronically unloaded hearts. *Circulation 107*, 1176-82.

[25] Kaye, D. M, Hoshijima, M, & Chien, K. R. (2008). Reversing advanced heart failure by targeting Ca2+ cycling. *Annu. Rev. Med. 59*, 13-28.

[26] Terracciano, C. M, Harding, S. E, Adamson, D, et al. (2003). Changes in sarcolemmal Ca entry and sarcoplasmic reticulum Ca content in ventricular myocytes from patients with end-stage heart failure following myocardial recovery after combined pharmacological and ventricular assist device therapy. *Eur. Heart J. 24*, 1329-39.

[27] Dipla, K, Mattiello, J. A, Jeevanandam, V, et al. (1998). Myocyte recovery after mechanical circulatory support in humans with end-stage heart failure. *Circulation 97*, 2316-22.

[28] Heerdt, P. M, Holmes, J. W, Cai, B, et al. (2000). Chronic unloading by left ventricular assist device reverses contractile dysfunction and alters gene expression in end-stage heart failure. *Circulation 102*, 2713-19.

[29] Ogletree-hughes, M. L, Stull, L. B, Sweet, W. E, et al. (2001). Mechanical unloading restores beta-adrenergic responsiveness and reverses receptor downregulation in the failing human heart. *Circulation 104*, 881-86.

[30] Terracciano, C. M, Hardy, J, Birks, E. J, et al. (2004). Clinical recovery from end-stage heart failure using leftventricular assist device and pharmacological therapy corre-

lates with increased sarcoplasmic reticulum calcium content but not with regression of cellular hypertrophy. *Circulation 109*, 2263-65.

[31] Harding, J. D. Piacentino V III, Gaughan JP, et al. (2001). Electrophysiological alterations after mechanical circulatory support in patients with advanced cardiac failure. *Circulation 104*, 1241-47.

[32] Xydas, S, Rosen, R. S, Ng, C, et al. (2006). Mechanical unloading leads to echocardiographic, electrocardiographic, neurohormonal, and histologic recovery. *J. Heart Lung Transplant. 25*, 7-15.

[33] Soppa, G. K, Lee, J, Stagg, M. A, et al. (2008). Prolonged mechanical unloading reduces myofilament sensitivity to calcium and sarcoplasmic reticulum calcium uptake leading to contractile dysfunction. *J. Heart Lung Transplant. 27*, 882-89.

[34] Yacoub, M. H. (2001). A novel strategy to maximize the efficacy of left ventricular assist devices as a bridge to recovery. *Eur. Heart J. 22*, 534-40.

[35] Soppa, GK, & Smolenski, . . 2005. Effects of chronic administration of clenbuterol on function and metabolism of adult rat cardiac muscle. *Am. J. Physiol. Heart Circ. Physiol.* 288:H1468-76

[36] Birks, E. J, Tansley, P. D, Hardy, J, et al. (2006). Left ventricular assist device and drug therapy for the reversal of heart failure. *N. Engl. J. Med. 355*, 1873-84.

[37] Pagani, F. D, Miller, L. W, Russell, S. D, et al. (2009). Extended mechanical circulatory support with a continuous-flow rotary left ventricular assist device. *J. Am. Coll. Cardiol.* , 54, 312-21.

[38] Christiansen, S, Klocke, A, & Autschbach, R. (2008). Past, present, and future of long-term mechanical cardiac support in adults. *J. Card. Surg. 23*, 664-76.

[39] Lietz, K, Long, J. W, Kfoury, A. G, et al. Outcomes of left ventricular assist device implantation as destination therapy in the post-REMATCH era: implications for patient selection. *Circulation* (2007). , 116, 497-505.

[40] Katherine LietzM.D., Ph.D. Destination Therapy: Patient Selection and Current Outcomes; *J Card Surg* (2010). , 25, 462-471.

[41] Lars, H. Lund, Jennifer Matthews and Keith Aaronson et al.Patient selection for left ventricular assist devices. European Journal of Heart Failure ((2010).

[42] Sean, R. Wilson, MD; Gilbert H. Mudge Jr, MD; Garrick C. Stewart, MD; Michael M. Givertz, MD et al. Evaluation for a Ventricular Assist Device Selecting the Appropriate Candidate. Circulation (2009). , 119, 2225-2232.

[43] Piccione W JrLeft ventricular assist device implantation: short and long-term surgical complications. *J Heart Lung Transplant* (2000). S, 89-94.

[44] Birks, E. J, Tansley, P. D, Yacoub, M. H, et al. Incidence and clinical management of life threatening left ventricular assist device failure. *J Heart Lung Transplant* (2004). , 23, 964-9.

[45] Horton, S. C, Khodaverdian, R, Powers, A, et al. Left ventricular assist device malfunction: a systematic approach to diagnosis. *J Am Coll Cardiol* (2004). , 43, 1574-83.

[46] Scalia, G. M, Mccarthy, P. M, Savage, R. M, Smedira, N. G, & Thomas, J. D. Clinical utility of echocardiography in the management of implantable ventricular assist devices. *J Am Soc Echocardiogr* (2000). , 13, 754-63.

[47] Pae, W. E, Connell, J. M, Boehmer, J. P, et al. Neurologic events with a totally implantable left ventricular assist device: European LionHeart Clinical Utility Baseline Study (CUBS). *J Heart Lung Transplant* (2007). , 26, 1-8.

[48] Thomas, C. E, Jichici, D, Petrucci, R, Urrutia, V. C, & Schwartzman, R. J. Neurologic complications of the Novacor left ventricular assist device. *Ann Thorac Surg* (2001). , 72, 1311-5.

[49] Lazar, R. M, Shapiro, P. A, Jaski, B. E, et al. Neurological events during long-term mechanical circulatory support for heart failure: the Randomized Evaluation of Mechanical Assistance for the Treatment of Congestive Heart Failure (REMATCH) experience. *Circulation* (2004). , 109, 2423-7.

[50] Tsukui, H, Abla, A, Teuteberg, J. J, et al. Cerebrovascular accidents in patients with a ventricular assist device. *J Thorac Cardiovasc Surg* (2007). , 134, 114-23.

[51] Slaughter, M. S, Sobieski, M. A, Gallagher, C, Dia, M, & Silver, M. A. Low incidence of neurologic events during long-term support with the HeartMate XVE left ventricular assist device. *Tex Heart Inst J* (2008). , 35, 245-9.

[52] Gordon, R. J, Quagliarello, B, & Lowy, F. D. Ventricular assist device related infections. *Lancet Infect Dis* (2006). , 6, 426-37.

[53] Simon, D, Fischer, S, Grossman, A, et al. Left ventricular assist device-related infection: treatment and outcome. *Clin Infect Dis* (2005). , 40, 1108-15.

[54] Zierer, A, Melby, S. J, Voeller, R. K, et al. Late-onset driveline infections: the Achilles' heel of prolonged left ventricular assist device support. *Ann Thorac Surg* (2007). , 84, 515-20.

[55] Gordon, S. M, Schmitt, S. K, Jacobs, M, et al. Nosocomial bloodstreaminfections in patients with implantable left ventricular assist devices. *Ann Thorac Surg* (2001). , 72, 725-30.

[56] Holman, W. L, Park, S. J, Long, J. W, et al. Infection in permanent circulatory support: experience from the REMATCH trial. *J Heart Lung Transplant* (2004). , 23, 1359-65.

[57] Chinn, R, Dembitsky, W, Eaton, L, et al. Multicenter experience: prevention and management of left ventricular assist device infections. *Asaio J* (2005). , 51, 461-70.

[58] Nurozler, F, Argenziano, M, Oz, M. C, & Naka, Y. Fungal left ventricular assist device endocarditis. *Ann Thorac Surg* (2001). , 71, 614-8.

[59] Jerry, D, Estep, M. D, Raymond, F, Stainback, M. D, Stephen, H, & Little, M. D. Guillermo Torre, MD,* William A. Zoghbi, MD*et al. The Role of Echocardiography and Other Imaging Modalities in Patients With Left Ventricular Assist Devices. J Am Coll Cardiol Img. (2010). , 3(10), 1049-1064.

[60] Foray, A, Williams, D, Reemtsma, K, Oz, M, & Mancini, D. Assessment of submaximal exercise capacity in patients with left ventricular assist devices. Circulation (1996). II, 222-6.

[61] Anker, S. D, Chua, T. P, Ponikowski, P, et al. Hormonal changes and catabolic/anabolic imbalance in chronic heart failure and their importance for cardiac cachexia. Circulation (1997). , 96, 526-34.

[62] Dang, N. C, Topkara, V. K, Kim, B. T, Lee, B. J, Remoli, R, & Naka, Y. Nutritional status in patients on left ventricular assist device support. J Thorac Cardiovasc Surg (2005). e, 3-4.

Chapter 2

Echocardiography and Hemodynamic Monitoring Tools for Clinical Assessment of Patients on Mechanical Circulatory Support

Sabino Scolletta, Bonizella Biagioli,
Federico Franchi and Luigi Muzzi

Additional information is available at the end of the chapter

http://dx.doi.org/10.5772/55918

1. Introduction

Mechanical circulatory support (MCS) has become an essential part of the treatment strategy for patients suffering acute, reversible ventricular dysfunction or end-stage heart failure. Cardiac function and systemic blood flow monitoring in patients on ventricular assist device (VAD) is essential in order to avoid low output syndrome, which remains one of the leading causes of death after MCS.

Echocardiography is considered as the procedure of choice for the evaluation of cardiac performance and to gather other critical information both in the pre, intra and postoperative phases. Also, echo-Doppler-based methods can be used to calculate the flow velocity and volume and hence systemic blood flow. Unfortunately, due to intrinsic nature, echocardiography cannot be considered a bedside continuous monitoring system.

Several methods are now available for blood flow assessment and cardiac output (CO) monitoring. An ideal hemodynamic monitoring system should comprise all the key factors listed in Table 1. However, such a system does not currently exist. Indeed, the ultrasonic flowmetry from the graft's outflow is considered as the gold standard method; however, its use is limited to the intraoperative period. The thermodilution continuous CO method is increasingly used. However, it incorporates a thermal coil integrated into the pulmonary artery catheter and it cannot be used in right VAD (RVAD) patients. Pulse contour methods derive systemic blood flow from the analysis of the arterial pressure waveform. They provide a fast response time and may represent suitable tools to assess CO and other hemodynamic variables in patients on MCS.

This chapter will review the most commonly used techniques to assess cardiac function and systemic blood flow in patients assisted with MCS.

1.1. Classification of MCS

Current devices for mechanical circulatory assistance provide a wide spectrum of support, ranging from short-term to intermediate and long-term duration [1,2], and the current indications for ventricular assist device implantation are: bridge to cardiac transplantation, bridge to recovery or destination therapy for patient not candidate to heart transplantation.

For these different purposes, different types of devices able to provide pulsatile or continuous blood flow are available for clinical use, and selection of MCS device mainly depends by the degree of the support required, the estimated duration of assistance, the invasiveness of the implantation procedure and the patient's need for postoperative mobility [3].

Over the years, three devices generations have succeeded and the rationale of the innovations and modifications has been mainly focused on decreasing the rate of complications, being the main determinant for patient outcome (chiefly thromboembolisms, bleeding, mechanical failure and infections).

1.1.1. First-generation devices

The first generation devices (Thoratec paracorporeal ventricular assist device and Abiomed BVS 5000) were largely used for bridge to transplant or bridge to recovery. They were able to provide pulsatile flow by means of large paracorporeal consoles but were associated with high mortality and complication rates [4,5]. Nevertheless when used for patients as bridge to transplantation, survival to transplant improved and resulted in optimizing patients' overall hemodynamic status allowing them to be better surgical candidates [6].

1.1.2. Second-generation ventricular assist devices

The second-generation of devices (HeartMate IP/XVE, Novacorand Arrow Lionheart) also provided pulsatile flow but were implanted as intra-corporeal pumps allowing greater patient mobility and resulting in reduced complications and infection rates compared to first-generation devices [3].

1.1.3. Third-generation ventricular assist devices

The concept and the goal of destination therapy guided the development of third-generation VADs (HeartMate II, Berlin Incor, MicroMed Debakey and Jarvik 2000) [3].

The clinical objectives of destination therapy VADs are to restore an adequate blood flow, preserving end-organ function and providing significant decompression of failing ventricle [7] virtually restoring a normal resting hemodynamics, exercise tolerance and normalizing metabolic as well as neuro-humoral functions [2].

Such devices are currently used and explored in clinical practice. They are fully implantable axial flow pumps, with design modifications (i.e., lack of percutaneous lines and implantation within the pericardium avoiding the need for a pump pocket) that will decrease patient's complications [8].

1.2. Hemodynamic principles of VADs functioning: Basic concepts

VADs consist of electromechanical pumps usually placed in parallel with the native patient's circulation. Their principal components consist in:

1. *Inflow cannula*. Direct the blood from one of the heart chambers to the device. Typically, for a LVAD, the inflow cannula originates in the left atrium (LA) or left ventricle (LV). For a RVAD, the inflow cannula originates in the right atrium (RA) or right ventricle (RV).

2. *Pump*. Provides propulsion to the blood. The generated flow can be either pulsatile (pneumatically or electromechanically driven pumps, e.g., Abiomed BVS 5000, HeartMate I, Novacor, Thoratec), or continuous such as in the most recent axial-flow devices (HeartMate II, Jarvik 2000, MicroMed DeBakey, Berlin Incor Heart) [9-11] or centrifugal pumps (Biomedicus, Levitronix-Centrimag and TandemHeart) [12,13]. Because of the larger size, the requirement of unidirectional valves in the VAD inflow and outflow cannulas, and complicated control mechanism of pulsatile VADs, axial flow pumps have been gaining popularity [11]. In non-pulsatile axial-flow pumps, the propulsion principle is based on a rotating impeller pump, which ejects blood to the systemic circulation at a fixed rate depending on pump speed and inflow–outflow pressure gradient. The advantages of these systems are that they are smaller, do not require unidirectional valves, are more durable, and typically generate higher flows at lower pressures.

3. *Outflow cannula*. The outflow cannula returns the blood to the patient. The LVAD outflow cannula is usually anastomosed to the ascending aorta (or descending aorta with Jarvik 2000) and to the main pulmonary artery (PA) in RVAD.

4. *Controller*. The controller operates the pump by receiving and processing information from it.

Different devices and controllers range from paracorporeal VADs with transcutaneous inflow and outflow cannulas or intracorporeal VADs with transcutaneous drivelines, to completely implantable intra- or extra-ventricular systems. The VAD performance characteristics produce distinctive relationships between pressure and flow in the circulation. These will determine measured hemodynamic parameters as well as echocardiographic signals (such as the continuous (CW) and pulsed wave (PW) Doppler signals) [5,14].

2. Echocardiography in patients assisted with VAD

Since low-output syndrome with impaired tissue perfusion and organ dysfunction still remains the main cause of death in such patients [15,16], the determination of both left ventricular function and CO is a decisive and mandatory issue in all the patients implanted with VAD. Echocardiography is the principal tool to investigate the LV function whereas different methods are available for CO estimation. Nonetheless, because of changes in hemodynamic and blood flow physiology related to every single device, the type of generated blood flow (pump type) and the position of cannulas and pump, respect to native patient's circulation, make the evaluation of CO and ventricular function a challenging issue.

2.1. Echocardiographic examination

Echocardiography is an important tool in the management of patients undergoing VAD implantation, since it can easily provide critical information about pre-operative anatomic abnormalities, guide the device implantation procedure, and evaluate post-insertion cardiac and device function. Combined information from both transthoracic (TTE) and transesophageal (TEE) echocardiography are used pre, intra and postoperatively to this purpose [17].

Echocardiographic assessment of patients undergoing VAD insertion involves aspects pertaining both to a general echocardiographic examination and to specific considerations associated with the VAD. The variety of VAD models with different basic and operational principles actually impose specific echocardiographic assessment targeted to the characteristics of the implanted device. This makes essential that the sonographer have a clear understanding of the specific device characteristics to perform a suitable examination. In addition to the standard assessment, essential device-specific considerations in the echocardiographic evaluation include:

a. *pre-VAD examination*. This includes the analysis of the heart and large vessels to exclude significant abnormalities, such as aortic regurgitation, tricuspid regurgitation, mitral stenosis, pulmonic regurgitation, patent foramen ovale, or other pathologies leading to right-to-left shunt after LVAD insertion. Moreover, intracardiac thrombi, ventricular scars, pulmonary hypertension, pulmonary embolism, and atherosclerotic disease in the ascending aorta can be easily detected by TTE.

b. *intra- and post-VAD examination*. The examination includes the device function evaluation and reassessment of the heart and large vessels. The examination of the device is focused to confirm the effective device and heart deairing, the cannulas or device alignment and patency, and competency of device valves using two-dimensional, color, continuous and pulsed wave Doppler modalities. Heart reassessment must provide information to exclude aortic regurgitation and intracardiac right-to-left shunt, as well as to assess the RV function, LV unloading, and the effect of device settings respect to global heart function.

2.2. Defects creating intracardiac shunts

2.2.1. *Patent Foramen Ovale(PFO) and other abnormalities of interatrial septum*

The presence of PFO must be always ascertained before and after cardiopulmonary bypass (CPB). Because of increased LA pressure with rightward deviation of the interatrial septum in patients with LV failure, investigation of a PFO with color-Doppler echocardiography in the pre-CPB period can be easily performed (demonstrating a left-to-right shunt). Conversely a bubble study may not reveal a PFO due to the difficulty in producing a reversal of the left-to-right atrial pressure gradient in the presence of left heart failure. Likewise, in the case of biventricular failure, increased RA and LA pressures reduce the interatrial pressure gradient, hindering PFO detection by both agitated saline and color-Doppler. It must be always kept in mind that patients without a detected PFO in the pre-CPB examination can present it once LVAD becomes operating, because the LV unloading and decreased LA pressure associated with maintained/increased right heart pressures, may open an unsealed PFO. Those hemodynamic conditions can favour a paradoxical embolism. Because the presence of right-to left shunt can result in the development of severe hypoxemia (with the degree of shunting also aggravated by chest closure resulting in RA pressure increase), significant right-to-left shunting should always be assessed with TEE as early as possible and also during the weaning from CPB, because a PFO can be potentially detected even before complete separation. Early detection is fundamental because the presence of a PFO requires return to CPB for closure.

2.2.2. *Valvular and ascending aortic defects*

2.2.2.1. *Aortic valve opening and function*

Because of the increased aortic-LV pressure gradient the aortic valve (native or prosthetic) usually remain closed throughout the whole cardiac cycle during full LVAD assistance. This is typical for pulsatile VADs generating full CO. Conversely, in VADs providing partial or intermittent unloading (e.g., Jarvik 2000, HeartMate II) [18] a transient opening of the aortic valve might be detected. In such devices the intermittent opening of the aortic valve is a target for device setting (e.g., opening of the aortic valve documented echocardiographically once every three cardiac cycles for a HeartMate II and reduction of pump output in the Jarvik 2000 to allow for ventricular ejection through the aortic valve) [5]. In these cases M-mode imaging is used to assess the duration of aortic valve opening [5]. In some particular devices, such as the Impella (that is placed in trans-aortic position) TEE examination is fundamental for its correct positioning.

The identification of aortic regurgitation (AR) (either pre- or postoperative) is essential in patients implanted with a LVAD. Indeed, AR may reduce the forward stroke volume generated by the LVAD as a consequence of a blood back-flow (LVAD ejected blood) into the LV. However, some aspects make the pre-operative echocardiographic evaluation of AR challenging in patients suffering severe heart failure because the combination of increased LV end-diastolic pressure and low aortic diastolic pressure (lowered transvalvular gradient) may underestimate the degree of AR [19]. The actual rate of late AR (not pre-existent to LVAD implantation) is relatively low and some recognized factors may contribute to its development during LVAD support, such as the presence of a closed native valve exposed to systolic pressure (rather than diastolic) [20], and VAD cannula in the ascending aorta determining valve distortion.

Other mechanisms of late AR include endocarditis [21], aortic dissection [22,23], and aortic leaflet prolapse or perforation.

Nevertheless the presence of severe or moderate AR usually mandate the surgical correction [24] consisting alternatively in simple leaflets closure (patients requiring long-term support, bridge to transplantation) which may prevent from systemic embolization also [19,25] or aortic valve replacement/repair (patients candidate to short-term support, bridge to recovery).

Differently from AR, aortic stenosis (AS) does not determine particular problems in patients receiving a LVAD because the systemic blood flow is mainly dependent from the pump output respect to residual ventricular ejection. This is particular true for pulsatile LVADs that are able to provide a full cardiac unloading. However in the case of VADs providing a partial or intermittent ventricular unloading (axial flow devices, with intermittent aortic valve opening) the presence of AS could conversely affect the total systemic blood flow. For this reason patient with pre-existent AS are not considered as the ideal candidates for such kind of devices. As for AR the development of aortic stenosis after LVAD implantation, particularly in long term support with pulsatile devices can result from commissural fusion [26], progressive thrombosis of the aortic valve [27] (due to blood stagnation, low level of anticoagulation, limited/absent aortic valve movement during LVAD function).

2.2.2.2. *Ascending aorta*

Pre and intraoperative examination of the ascending aorta is mandatory in patients receiving a LVAD since it must detect calcifications, atherosclerotic plaques or any other abnormality of the vessel in the site of anastomosis of the outflow cannula. Depending from VAD's outflow cannula placement site the descending aorta should be assessed with the same goal (e.g.,Jarvik 2000). Atherosclerotic plaques of ≥5 mm and/or protruding and/or mobile components are associated with increased risk of cerebral embolic events.

2.2.2.3. *Tricuspid regurgitation*

Tricuspid Regurgitation (TR) is common in patients affected by heart failure [28]. However the presence of an adequate RV function (to maintain an adequate blood flow to the left heart for LVAD filling) is the key of success in patients receiving a LVAD. In this scenario a significant postoperative TR can negatively affect the RV function with possible development of a low output syndrome.

Echocardiographic evaluation of the tricuspid valve (TV) is affected by RV contractility, preload and afterload of RA, preload and afterload of RV.

Ventricular enlargement, due to preload and afterload increase, contributes to the development of tricuspid regurgitation (annulus dilation and chordal tension) [20,29]. The reduction of right ventricle preload (pulmonary artery pressure) in patient on LVAD actually does not determine a reduction of post-operative TR which can, conversely and most frequently, worsen after implantation.

Different factors and mechanisms are responsible for acute worsening of TR, such as increased RV preload due to an increased left-sided output delivered by a functioning, increased PA pressure and RV dysfunction due to the inflammatory response to surgery, CPB and blood transfusion, and leftward shift of the interventricular septum produced by the LVAD unloading and favoured by hypovolemia and high VAD flows.

The influence of LVAD settings on the degree of TR by shifting the interventricular septum can be frequently observed in axial flow devices where excessively high flow settings exacerbate TR, presumably by mechanisms such as distraction of the septal papillary muscle with systolic restriction of septal leaflet motion and distortion of the tricuspid annulus. Relative RV overload and increased PA pressures can further contribute to worsened TR.

Echocardiography must guide the diagnosis of TR and determine the functional cause and mechanism which, once identified, should be minimized by adjusting the pump setting (flow reduction flow) in order to reduce the degree of regurgitation and consequently improve RV function.

2.2.2.4. Mitral regurgitation / stenosis

Mitral Regurgitation (MR) in end-stage heart failure and cardiomyopathy is common [28,30] and it mostly consists in a functional pathology due to an incomplete leaflet coaptation secondary to a negative remodeling of both the LV (increased sphericity and dilation, apical displacement of the papillary muscles with typical valve tethering) and mitral annulus (increased intertrigonal and anterior-posterior annular size).

The reduction of LV size after LVAD implantation, differently from TR, almost always contributes to ameliorate mitral leaflets coaptation and, thus, to reduce the degree of pre-exixtent regurgitation. For this reason, the finding of MR pre-VAD rarely indicates surgical correction.

Conversely, the persistence of significant MR may indicate suboptimal ventricular unloading during LVAD support. During VAD support with pulsatile devices MR can, however, contribute to patient's symptoms and, in some instances, indicate the surgical correction. Actually the asynchronous pulsation of the VAD and the assisted ventricle can determine/worsen mitral regurgitation when LV contraction occurs against both the closed aortic and the inflow VAD valve.

A low output syndrome during LVAD assistance can result from the presence of mitral stenosis (MS) resulting in reduced pump filling. Moreover chronic MS associated with pulmonary hypertension can contribute to postoperative RV dysfunction. Thus, the presence of MS should be always evaluated in the planning of LVAD insertion and critical MS surgically treated at the same time.

2.2.2.5. Pulmonic valve

Although rare, the presence of pulmonary valve lesions may have important consequences on the RV function and output. Critical pulmonic stenosis (PS) in patients under LVADs can determine an important pressure overload in the RV, compromising the RV output both directly and indirectly by contributing to RV failure. With regard to pulmonic insufficiency (PI) apply the same considerations given for aortic regurgitation in the case of RVAD (reduced forward flow) while in patients under LVAD the presence of PI (moderate or greater) may contribute to RV overload/dilatation and possible TR determining a dysfunction of the RV.

2.3. Ventricular assessment

2.3.1. Right ventricle

LVAD assistance can result in two possible and opposite effects on the RV function. The afterload reduction caused by the left-sided pump may positively increase the function of the right ventricle. Opposite, the contemporary augmented left output resulting in increased preload for the right heart sections can be detrimental in the presence of a compromised RV function which can rapidly decompensate [31]. The leftward septal shifts also favour RV dysfunction by reducing RV global contractility [32,33]. Nevertheless, because the LVAD output is strictly dependent on preload, a sufficient RV function must be warranted to avoid a low output syndrome due to LVAD low flow.

As a result, the evaluation of pre-implant RV function and early post-operative detection of severe RV dysfunction (ranging from 9% to 33 in different series) play a key role for the success of LVAD assistance and patient's outcome because in the presence of severe RV failure placement of RVAD may be required and the earlier the detection and the RVAD insertion the better the outcome [34].

Despite a strong association between preoperative impaired RV function (low PA pressure, RV stroke work index) and need for RVAD placement has been demonstrated [35,36] RV failure following LVAD implantation in single patients still remains hard to be predicted because of the multiple factors potentially contributing to its development [35]. A thorough pre-operative evaluation of RV function and identification of any predictors for RV dysfunction is fundamental to select the patient's optimal device and to schedule each one for uni- or bi-ventricular support [35].

Echocardiography is a fundamental diagnostic tool to this purpose. Two-dimensional evaluation of the RV function and dimensions is made by analysing RV inflow–outflow in mid-esophageal (ME) view and the four-chamber views at transgastric level. This allows the assessment of both the longitudinal function (RV base-apex motion and free-wall motion) [37]. Quantitative measurements (global RV fractional area change [14,38], regional fractional area change [33], and the maximum derivative of the RV pressure (dP/dt max)) can be also used to detail the systolic function of the RV [39,40]. Analysis of tricuspid valve inflow profile is used for the assessment of diastolic dysfunction. Possible predictors of RV dysfunction after LVAD implantation are preoperative RV dilatation and increased preload and afterload, and RV fractional area change < 20%.

2.3.2. Left ventricle

Patients candidate to VAD insertion show a depressed LV function with a LV ejection fraction (LVEF) usually < 25%. The presence of severe LV dysfunction, particularly if associated with aneurismal apical dilatation increases the risk of apical clot formation. Pre-insertion evaluation

http://dx.doi.org/10.5772/55918

of the presence of thrombus in the site of inflow cannula/pump (Jarvik 2000) insertion is a crucial and mandatory issue of the echocardiographic examination.

Depending by the leading cause of heart failure, the ventricle dimensions and volumes can be normal or, more often, augmented.

Once on LVAD assistance, the ventricular unloading usually associates with a normalization of ventricular dimensions and volumes and complete unloading associates with no residual ventricular ejection and persistent closure of the aortic valve.

Echocardiographic "signs" of LVAD malfunction to be considered are spontaneous contrast in the LA or LV. Another important feature to be evaluated is the aspect of the interventricular septum (IVS) because a not adequately unloaded ventricle will show a rightward IVS deviation suggesting a possible insufficient pump output (due to pump failure, cannulas obstruction, or other causes).

Leftward IVS shift usually seen with rotary LVAD will, conversely, suggest an excessive ventricular decompression, which may associate to low pump output as well. Such event can be due to elevated pump speed, in an axial VAD, RV dysfunction or hypovolemia.

It is important to outline that because of ventricular unloading, the correct evaluation of systolic function is critical and not easy to be ascertained while on VAD assistance. Several echocardiographic indexes as well as hemodynamic measurements are used in clinical practice when patients are scheduled for possible weaning from VAD assistance (see text).

More recently the speckle tracking echocardiography has emerged as a new technique for the evaluation of myocardial function. This sophisticated method allows the analysis of longitudinal, radial and circumferential myocardial deformation (strain) providing a in-depth evaluation of both global and regional myocardial contractility. Moreover, speckle tracking echocardiography allows the evaluation of rotational and torsional dynamics of left ventricle function that only with magnetic resonance imaging (MRI) could be otherwise assessed.

2.4. Assessment of VAD components

2.4.1. VAD cannulas

VAD cannulas are made of woven polyester fabric having hyperechoic density in the echocardiographic imaging. Depending on single device characteristics, alternative cannulation methods are used leading to distinct echocardiographic images and considerations.

2.4.1.1. Inflow cannula (Jarvik 2000-pump)

The inflow cannulas correct positioning can be easily visualized on two-dimensional echocardiography although the precise three-dimensional visualization needs to alternative views (ME four-chamber for deviations towards the interventricular septum, ME two-chamber long-axis view to assess the anterior–posterior direction). In LVAD they can be placed either in LA or LV apex. When positioned in the apex it is important to verify that it is correctly aligned with the left ventricle inflow tract, facing the mitral valve opening without touching any wall of the ventricle. Colour-Doppler is a useful adjunct, since an accurately positioned cannula will show a unidirectional/laminar flow directed to the device, while the finding of turbulent flow will suggest a not appropriate placement or obstruction of the cannula (thrombosis or partial obstruction of the cannula by the ventricular wall). Device stroke volume and total blood flow can be evaluated by PW Doppler measurements obtained from both the inflow and outflow cannulas. By evaluating the RV and LV outflow tracts, flows PW Doppler can give also an estimation of eventual residual ventricular ejection in VADs providing only partial circulatory support.

2.4.1.2. Outflow cannula

In the most of the cases the ouflow cannula of LVADs is anastomosed, as an end-to-side anastomosis, in the right anterolateral portion of the ascending aorta. Other type of devices, (e.g., Jarvik 2000), may have the outflow cannula anastomosed either to the ascending aorta or to the descending thoracic aorta. A long axis view of the ascending aorta will usually show the outflow cannula anastomosis to the ascending aorta. In the case of RVAD the outflow cannula is usually positioned in the main pulmonary artery trunk (directly, or inserted through an incision in the RV apex) although the right PA the can be alternatively used. It can be easily visualized by two-dimensional echocardiography with a mid-esophageal 20–70° view. The flow patterns of the outflow cannulas can be evaluated with color-PW and CW-Doppler.

2.4.1.3. Devices with alternative principles and implantation techniques (Jarvik 2000)

Because new devices with alternative principles and cannulation methods have been introduced in the clinical practice particular echocardiographic evaluations and considerations are required.

Axial flow pumps offers a number of advantages respect to pulsatilepumps. They are relatively easy to be implanted (also without the use of CPB), they are smaller (producing a continuous unidirectional blood flow no valve are needed and do not require a compliance chamber for systolic-diastolic phases) and suitable for a wide size-range of patients and have lower rates of complications.

The Jarvik 2000 is an axial flow-based device implanted in the apex of the LV. Because it has no inflow cannula but the pump itself is positioned inside the left ventricle the TEE examination is important during and after implantation of this type of device.

It is mandatory that the sonographer is able to guide the precise coring position centred at the apex and, once implanted inside the ventricle, verify that the pump is perfect in axial alignment with the mitral valve.

Because no integrated flow sensors are available, echocardiographic evaluation is critical to assess the device performance and the global hemodynamic. Thus, after Jarvik200 implantation the degree of ventricular assistance/unloading (to achieve a full or partial assistance) must be evaluated by first establishing the speed range at which the aortic valve does not open (complete unloading). Then by progressively reducing the pump rotationsper minute (usually 1000 rpm steps) it must be assessed the speed at which the aortic valve opens.

Because outflow cannula of Jarvik 2000 is conventionally anastomosed (trans-pericardial) to the descending aorta flow patterns proximal and distal to the anastomotic site are quite different respect to VADs whose outflow cannula is placed in the ascending aorta. Particularly, at high device flows, which determine a complete unloading with permanent closure of the aortic valve, stagnation of blood in the ascending aorta and sinuses of Valsalva might occur with possible thrombosis and obstruction of the coronary ostia with detrimental consequences.

This risk must be reduced or eliminated with the intermittent reduction of the device output to allow ventricular ejection and phasic aortic valve opening which must be echocardiographycally assessed, since the degree of the outflow graft pulsatility alone do not predict the presence of systolic aortic valve opening [41].

2.4.1.4. Deairing

Intraoperative echocardiography is very useful for detection of micro- or macro-bubbles and result fundamental to direct de-airing of the heart after VAD implantion.

VADs components can contain significant amounts of air and, in adjunct, pulsatile devices using negative filling pressures may drag air from the thoracic cavity into the circulation especially at the inflow cannula insertion site resulting in the passage of air bubbles to the heart and systemic circulation. The most common locations to which air will migrate, once CPB is interrupted and pulmonary perfusion re-established, are the right coronary artery and the innominate artery possibly contributing to ventricular dysfunction and/or neurologic injury.

Careful deairing should be performed before aortic cross clamp removal and before the pump is set fully operational. Structures to be inspected include heart chambers and both ascending and descending aorta using different TEE views (ME aortic valve long-axis view, ME ascending aorta long-axis view and descending aorta short- and long-axis view).

2.5. Recovery and weaning

Identification of the ideal candidates for successful LVAD or RVAD weaning is still an open topic and object of current study. The decision about possibility of successful weaning depends on integration of clinical, hemodynamic and echocardiographic factors [42,43] as documented by several studies reporting recovery and weaning protocols based on cardiopulmonary testing, hemodynamic and echocardiographic variables [44].

The largest reports of weaning and removal from chronic LVAD support suggest as parameters indicative of myocardial recovery a left ventricular ejection fraction ≥40% and a left ventricular end diastolic diameter (LVEDD) inferior to 55-60mm [45]. Other echocardiographic variables indicative of left myocardial recovery may be considered the fractional area change > 40%, and the improved ventricular contractility.

Serial echocardiographic examination of the aortic valve opening movements, LVEF and diameters at every reduction step of support is essential to evaluate a possible weaning, because they will reflect the LV response to the progressive increase of preload and, thus, its actual recovery.

Invasive hemodynamic monitoring during dobutamine stress echocardiography has been also proposed as a clinical test to assess the response of the assisted ventricle to unloading and consider a possible weaning from assistance [46]. The improvement of cardiac index, LVEF in absence of increased LVEDD and pulmonary capillary wedge pressure ≤ 15 mm are considered favourable for successful device explantation.

The most important parameters to be evaluated and considered for weaning from RVAD assistance are the right ventricular function, the central venous pressure, the degree tricuspid regurgitation and the resulting left ventricular filling.

However, the evaluation and management of pulmonary vascular resistances (PVR) is the most crucial issue when trying to wean patients from RVAD assistance. Because the success of the procedure is actually strictly dependent by PVR optimization[47] when fixed PVR are present patients will need supplementary management before attempting the weaning. Echocardiographic and hemodynamic monitoring demonstrating left and right heart sections maintaining a good function while decreasing the pump assistance without elevation of the central venous pressure, and PVR indicate the possibility to successfully wean the patient from the RVAD support.

Echocardiography evaluation of PVR can be performed by using the following formula :

$PVR = (V_{max}TR / VTI_{RVOT}) + 0.16$. (PVR are expressed in Wood units; $V_{max}TR$= maximal tricuspid regurgitation velocity; VTI_{RVOT} = systolic velocity time integral of the RV outflow tract).

2.6. Echocardiography for systemic blood flow assessment

Echocardiography allows measurement of CO using standard two-dimensional imaging or, more commonly, Doppler-based methods.

Doppler-based methods apply the following principle: if an ultrasound beam is directed along the aorta using a probe, part of the ultrasound signal will be reflected back by the moving red blood cells at a different frequency. The resultant Doppler shift in the frequency can be used to calculate the flow velocity and volume and hence CO. In patients on MCS, LVAD- and RVAD-CO can be separately assessed with a simple procedure [48].

Left and right ventricular outflow tract velocity-time integrals (VTIs) can be obtained by pulse wave Doppler signals and used to estimate both the left and right stroke volume (SV) and cardiac output (CO). For reliable measurements care must be taken to ensure an optimal angle between the blood flow and Doppler beam. Once obtained the two (right and left) estimations of cardiac output the following formula is used to have an indirect measure of the VAD output: LVAD CO = (RVOT CO) – (LVOT CO).

A direct measurement of the VAD output can be also obtained using both the cross-sectional area and pulse wave Doppler derived VTI in the outflow graft. For such calculation, as previously mentioned, is necessary that the outflow graft blood flow and the Doppler beam are maintained aligned and parallel as much as possible. Is usually advisable to use both the direct and indirect method for CO estimations and verify their correlation because possible discrepancies can derive from incorrect probe alignment as well as overestimations of the graft's cross-sectional area, or the LVOT and RVOT diameters [41].

2.6.1. Echocardiography: Advantages and disadvantages

Echo-Doppler has the key advantage of providing additional variables in addition to blood flow as previously described. The main disadvantage of Echo-Doppler evaluation is that it is operator dependent and continuous measurement of CO using this technique is not possible. Moreover, Echo-Doppler evaluation may be applied either trans-thoracically or trans-esophageally, but the former does not always yields good images. On the other hand, trans-esophageal technique is more invasive and is uncomfortable in non-intubated patients.

Echo-Doppler CO estimates require a certain expertise, so that blood flow measurements may vary considerably due to the difficulty in assessment of the velocity time integral, calculation error due to the angle of insonation, and problems with correct measurement of the cross-sectional area. Conversely, smaller trans-esophageal Doppler probes than for standard esophageal echocardiography techniques may be inserted nasally. They are operator-independent, less invasive and better tolerated. However these probes focus on blood flow into the descending thoracic aorta, thus a reliable measurement of the total CO could not be provided [49]. (See Table 1 for the main advantages and disadvantages of echocardiography).

3. Thermodilution methods to assess cardiac output

The determination of cardiac output (CO) during MCS is crucial, as low-output syndrome is the main cause of death in such patients [15]. Several methods are available for blood flow estimation and CO monitoring. However, the hemodynamic changes subsequent to VAD implantation somehow limit the application of current methods for CO determination [50]. Two principal methods capable of assessing systemic blood flow are available in clinical practice: thermodilution (ThD) and transpulmonary ThD system.

3.1. Pulmonary thermodilution method

The techniques based on pulmonary ThD method employ a pulmonary artery catheter (PAC) to monitor CO. The intermittent ThD technique employs a bolus of ice-cold fluid, which is injected into the right atrium via a PAC. The change in temperature detected in the blood of the pulmonary artery is used to calculate CO. This technique is still widely considered as the standard method in clinical practice and it is taken as the reference approach when comparing new CO monitoring technologies [51]. More recently, PAC has been adapted to incorporate a thermal filament (Vigilance™, Edwards Life Sciences, Irvine, CA, USA) or thermal coil (OptiQ™, ICU Medical, San

Clemente, CA, USA) that warms blood in the superior vena cava and measures changes in blood temperature at the PAC tip using a thermistor [52]. These modified techniques provide continuous monitoring of systemic blood flow (continuous ThD-CO) and the displayed values represent an average of CO values over the previous 8-10 minutes.

3.2. Transpulmonary thermodilution method

The techniques based on transpulmonary thermodilution method allow CO to be assessed less invasively, using a central venous (to allow injection of the indicator) and an arterial catheter, rather than needing to introduce a catheter into the pulmonary artery. Among these systems, PiCCO (Pulsion Medical Systems, Munich, Germany), and LiDCO (LiDCO Ltd, London, UK) are the most widely used devices, which apply the same basic principles of dilution to monitor blood flow as with PAC thermodilution [53].

PiCCO uses injections of cold intravenous fluid as the indicator, measuring change in temperature downstream to estimate systemic blood flow [54]. LiDCO uses small amounts of lithium chloride as the indicator and measures levels using a lithium-selective electrode [55].

3.3. Pulmonary and transpulmonary thermodilution method: Advantages and disadvantages

The PAC has a key advantage over other systems in that it provides measurements of other hemodynamic parameters in addition to systemic blood flow, including pulmonary artery pressures, right-sided and left-sided filling pressures, and mixed venous oxygen saturation (SvO2). Moreover, the PiCCO system provides variables in addition to blood flow, such as global end-diastolic volume and measurements of extravascular lung water. All the aforementioned parameters are of importance in patients on MCS in order to improve treatment of pulmonary hypertension, avoid fluid overloading, hypo-oxygenation, and high oxygen consumption [18].

Another main advantage of continuous ThD-CO is that it eliminates variability in CO estimates in the presence of arrhythmias. However, it has the disadvantage of not displaying real-time values, thus limiting its usefulness for assessing abrupt hemodynamic changes in patients with hemodynamic instability [48].

Methods based on "cold" pulmonary ThD (bolus ThD), as well as systems for continuous "hot" ThD (continuous ThD-CO) are theoretically suitable in patients assisted with a left VAD (LVAD) but are unreliable techniques for patients on RVAD due to "cold or hot" indicator loss bypassed by the pump from the right heart sections [56]. Similar limitations exist for systems based on transpulmonary ThD, which cannot be applied to any patient on MCS [RVAD, LVAD or biventricular assist devices (BiVAD)] unless modified set-up are used for application during isolated RVAD, as indicator loss would happen in both the right and left heart sections [50]. However, the ThD techniques measure the right heart CO, which is conditioned by the systemic venous return and by "total" left CO. Thus, they could actually provide the true

http://dx.doi.org/10.5772/55918

systemic blood flow in patients on LVAD [56]. (See Table 1 for the main advantages and disadvantages of thermodilution methods).

Assessment of:	Echocardiography	Thermodilution (PAC)	Pulse Contour Methods
- Left ventricular function	+	-	+
- Right ventricular function	+	+	-
- Anatomical features	+	-	-
- Cardiac output	+	+	+
- Systemic arterial pressure	-	-	+
- Pulmonary arterial pressure	+	+	-
- Systemic vascular resistances	-	+	+
- Pulmonary vascular resistances	+	+	-
- Preload	+	+	+/-
- Blood flow generated by VAD	+	-	+/-
- Cardiac valve function	+	-	-
- VAD components	+	-	-
- Mixed venous oxygen saturation	-	+	-
- Extravascular lung water		-	+/-
General requirements of an "ideal" tool			
- Accuracy	+	+	+/-
- Reproducibility	+	+	I
- Fast response time	-	-	+
- Operator independency	-	-	+
- Easy to use	-	+	+
- Continuous use	-	+/-	+
- Cost effectiveness	-	+	+/-
- Minimally invasive	+	-	+/-
- Clear data display and interpretation	+	+	+
- Neonates to adults	+	-	+/-
- Information that is able to guide therapy	+	+	+

+ satisfactory; - not satisfactory; +/- only some tools. PAC, pulmonary artery catheter.VAD, ventricular assist device.

Table 1. Main desirable characteristics of a monitoring tool to be used in patients on mechanical circulatory assistance (see text for details)

4. Pulse contour methods to estimate systemic blood flow

The analysis of the arterial trace is the key point of the so called "pulse contour methods" (PCMs). These techniques are based on the main assumption that the pressure rise during systole is related to the systolic filling of the aorta and proximal large arteries [57]. Thus, stroke volume, and hence CO, can be derived by means of the analysis of the shape of the arterial trace and the area under the pressure curve [58]. These are low-invasive techniques and allow beat-by-beat CO determinations. Indeed, these systems provide a fast response time and may represent suitable tools in patients on MCS, in whom sudden hemodynamic changes may lead to hypotension and low output syndrome.

There are presently four major PCMs that are able to calculate CO and other cardiovascular parameters from the analysis of the arterial pressure waveform: 1) PiCCO Monitor (Pulsion Medical Systems, Munich, Germany), 2) LiDCO System (LiDCO Ltd, London, UK), 3) Vigileo Monitor (Edwards Lifesciences LLC, Irvine, CA), and 4) MostCare Monitor (Vygon Health, Padua, Italy) [54].

The PiCCO needs transpulmonary thermodilution for its calibration (i.e., iced bolus in a central venous line) and a catheter into the femoral artery for the analysis of the arterial trace [59]. The LiDCO system measures systemic blood flow after an external calibration with an intravenous (centrally or peripherally) bolus of lithium [60]. The Vigileo system does not need external calibration with a bolus but it requires internal calibration (i.e., patient demographic and physical characteristics) for arterial impedance estimation [61]. The MostCare monitor has the innovative feature of not necessitating external or internal calibration, being based on PRAM (Pressure Recording Analytical Method) algorithm. Indeed, PRAM analyses the shape of the arterial trace taking into account all the points of the pressure wave. Simultaneously, it relates these points to the systolic and diastolic area under the pressure wave to estimate the interaction of left ventricle contraction with aortic impedance and compliance changes [62].

4.1. Pulse contour methods: Some practical considerations

Methods based on external calibration (i.e., bolus injected into a central or peripheral line) are unreliable techniques for patients on RVAD due to indicator loss bypassed by the VAD from the right heart sections [48]. Actually, these PCMs cannot be applied to any patient on MCS (RVAD, LVAD or biventricular assist devices (BiVAD)) as their external calibration is affected by indicator loss in both the right and left heart sections [63].

In order to avoid these limitations, PiCCO has been used in a patient on RVAD (Levitronix-CentriMag, Levitronix GmbH, Zurich, Switzerland) with a modified set-up for calibrating the system. Basically, the investigators positioned a left atrial catheter to inject the iced solution, instead of using a central venous catheter for the iced bolus [64]. However, this modified set-up cannot be used in clinical practise because it is very invasive and highly risky.

A modified set-up of lithium bolus dilution was used for the calibration of LiDCO in patients supported by a centrifugal pump (LevitronixCentriMag, Levitronix GmbH, Zurich, Switzerland) in the RVAD configuration (between the right atrium and pulmonary artery). Indeed, just before lithium bolus administration to the central venous catheter, the investigators increased the RVAD's revolutions per minute (RPM) as much as possible to ensure that all the blood flowed through the RVAD and to avoid RVAD suction events. The increase in RPM before calibration caused streamlined blood flow from the right atrium to the RVAD, excluding blood leakage through the native right ventricle [65].

MostCare has been recently used in 12 patients implanted with a pulsatile left ventricular assist device (LVAD) (HeartMate-I XVE, HM-I, Thoratec Corporation, Pleasanton, CA, USA) [48] and in one patient undergoing left (Jarvik 2000 axial flow pump, Jarvik Heart, Inc., New York, NY) and right (Levitronix CentriMag, Levitronix GmbH, Zurich, Switzerland) ventricular assist device implant [66]. Good performance with MostCare in such patients was found. Moreover, there was no need for changing the set-up of the device, as it is the only PCM that does not need external/internal calibration [66].

4.2. Pulse contour methods: Advantages, limitations and drawbacks in pulsatile and non-pulsatile VAD

Incomplete LV unloading during mechanical circulatory support can occur as the result of inadvertent and transient changes in afterload and preload (e.g. heart–lung interactions in patients who are mechanically ventilated). As a consequence, the native heart can unpredictably open the aortic valve and eject a variable amount of blood into the ascending aorta [48]. Moreover, when a pulsatile LVAD is set to operate in fixed-rate mode, independently of patient's heart rate, such a discrepancy can itself determine the occurrence of residual effective LV contractions and stroke outputs that can contribute to "total" CO (blood flow generated by the LVAD plus stroke volumes produced by the native heart). Thus, depending on the patient's heart rate and the device's stroke rate, arterial blood pressure waves related to ventricular ejection may coincide with LVAD arterial pulse waves (being unapparent) or may be variably interposed between the LVAD arterial pulse waves (Figure 1) [63].

A main advantage of PCMs is that they compute systemic blood flow from the analysis of a peripheral artery. Therefore, their blood flow estimation could represent the true systemic perfusion (i.e., the sum of the contributions from the native left ventricle ejecting through the aortic valve, and the pump ejecting directly into the aorta) [63].

A major limitation of PCMs resides in the fact that an arterial pulsatile pressure wave (i.e., pulse pressure) must be present for CO estimation. Thus, some issues about their reliability exist for non-pulsatile VADs, where incomplete LV unloading must occur to generate a pulse pressure sufficient to allow PCMs to compute CO. Conversely, with pulsatile VADs an arterial pulsatility can be anyhow detected, independently of ventricular loading or unloading conditions. In such conditions, uncalibrated PCMs should be able to analyse the arterial pressure wave morphology in any condition of LV preload [16].

With respect to pulsatile pump flow, rotary continuous-flow VADs produce less pulsatile and non-physiologic flows, and their hemodynamic characteristics are different from pulsatile VADs. First, at a given speed rotation, the flow through a rotary device is variable, generally unquantifiable and it is sensitive to the pressure gradient across it (aortic minus left ventricular pressure). Secondly, if the pump speed is too fast, the arterial pressure waveform decreases and the dicrotic notch is absent (indicating a closed aortic valve). Finally, with a rotary VAD, the fluctuations in left ventricular pressure are transmitted to the systemic arteries through the device even when the pump speed is sufficiently high to maintain the closure of the aortic valve. This may have important clinical consequences (e.g. aortic valve cusp fusion and thrombosis in the ascending aorta) [67]. PCMs could be useful under these circumstances, as PCMs analyse pulsatile flows and cannot work without a minimum pulse pressure. Indeed, a "no-value" alarm on the screen could serve as a "wake-up call" for an in-depth hemodynamic evaluation. This is particularly true for MostCare, which displays the dicrotic notch (and hence the aortic valve closure) at each cardiac cycle [68].

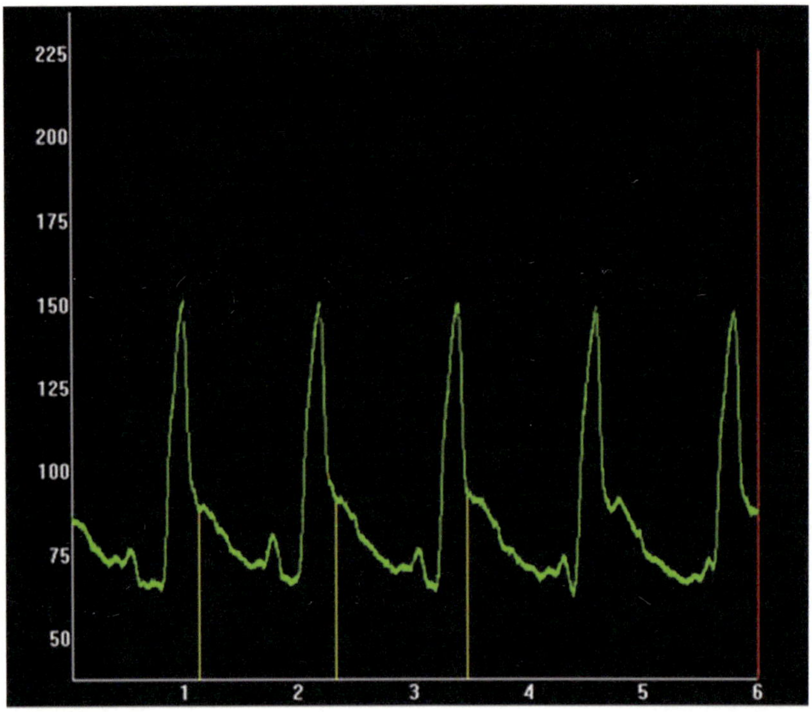

Figure 1. The figure 1 shows the arterial wave recording of a patient under pulsatile left ventricular assist device (LVAD) by the pulse contour method MostCare-PRAM (Pressure Recording Analytical Method). Values on y-axis are arterial pressures (mmHg). On x-axis are the cardiac cycles over time. The yellow vertical lines represent the identification of the dicrotic notch at each cardiac cycle. The arterial pressure waves are generated by LVAD stroke outputs. Of note, some smaller pressure waves are interposed between them. These smaller arterial traces represent residual left ventricular ejections of blood from the native heart. MostCare calculates the actual systemic total blood flow from the analysis of the sum of both the waves (i.e., stroke volumes produced by the artificial plus the native ventricle) (see text for details).

A major advantage of PCMs is that they can provide information on fluid responsiveness and cardiac function. In particular, MostCare is able to measure dP/dt (an index of myocardial contractility) and cardiac cycle efficiency (CCE, an index of ventricular-arterial coupling). Both these indices may have importance in the assessment of cardiovascular performance during the weaning from a VAD.

However, several factors could affect the accuracy of blood flow measurements and hemodynamic evaluation based on the analysis of the arterial waveform, such as arterial pathology in the proximal segments, vasoplegic patients on vasoconstrictor therapy. Indeed, all these conditions may affect the transmission of the pressure wave. Moreover, damped arterial waveforms and inadequate pulse detection (e.g., catheter dislodgement) may influence the precision of the pressure wave analysis [54,57,69,70]. (See Table 1 for the main advantages and disadvantages of pulse contour methods).

5. Conclusions

The development of mechanical circulatory support technology is now moving from displacement pumps (pulsatile flow) to axial and centrifugal pumps (continuous flow). Hemodynamic evaluation and measurement of blood flow is of crucial importance in patients on mechanical circulatory support.

Echocardiography has emerged as an important tool to assess hemodynamic performance in patients assisted with a ventricular assist device. However, it is operator dependent and cannot be used as a continuous bedside monitoring device. On the other hand, other hemodynamic monitoring techniques provide information on cardiac function and systemic blood flow on a beat-by-beat basis. Unfortunately, many of them they have the limitation of not being applicable in some circumstances.

An ideal hemodynamic monitoring system should comprise all the key factors listed in Table 1. However, such a system does not currently exist so we must try and choose devices that have a maximum of these attributes, bearing in mind that there is no "one size fits all" type of system and one should, therefore, select the system most appropriate for each patient and for each type of problem [54]. This is particularly true for patients supported with mechanical circulatory support, in whom abrupt hemodynamic changes may lead to severe arterial hypotension and clinical instability, which, in turn, are responsible for low output syndrome and poor outcome.

Author details

Sabino Scolletta*, Bonizella Biagioli, Federico Franchi and Luigi Muzzi

*Address all correspondence to: sabino.scolletta@unisi.it

Department of Medical Biotechnologies, Unit of Cardiac Surgery, Anesthesia and Intensive Care, S. Maria alle Scotte University Hospital, Siena, Italy

References

[1] Hetzer R, Muller JH, Weng YG, Loebe M, Wallukat G. Midterm follow-up of patients who underwent removal of a left ventricular assist device after cardiac recovery from end-stage dilated cardiomyopathy. J ThoracCardiovascSurg 2000;120:843–53.

[2] Leprince P, Combes A, Bonnet N, Ouattara A, Luyt CE, Theodore P, Leger P, Pavie A. Circulatory support for fulminant myocarditis: consideration for implantation, weaning and explantation. Eur J CardiothoracSurg 2003;24:399–403.

[3] Goldstein D, Oz M, Rose E. Implantable left ventricular assist devices. N Engl J Med 1998; 339:1522-1533.

[4] Kirklin JK, Holman WL. Mechanical circulatory support therapy as a bridge to transplant or recovery (new advances).CurrOpinCardiol 2006;21:120–6.

[5] Mitter N, Sheinberg R. Update on ventricular assist devices. CurrOpinAnaesthesiol 2010;23(1):57-66.

[6] Maybaum S, Williams M, Barbone A, Levin H, Oz M, Mancini D. Assessment of synchrony relationships between the native left ventricle and the HeartMate left ventricular assist device. J Heart Lung Transplant 2002;21:509–15.

[7] Joffe II, Jacobs LE, Lampert C, Owen AA, Ioli AW, Kotler MN. Role of echocardiography in perioperative management of patients undergoing open heart surgery. Am Heart J 1996;131:162–76.

[8] Park SJ, Tector A, Piccioni W, Raines E, Gelijns A, Moskowitz A, Rose E, Holman W, Furukawa S, Frazier OH, Dembitsky W. Left ventricular assist devices as destination therapy: a new look at survival. J ThoracCardiovascSurg 2005;129:9–17.

[9] Mihaylov D, Verkerke GJ, Rakhorst G. Mechanical circulatory support systems - a review. Technol Health Care 2000;8:251–66.

[10] Gemmato CJ, Forrester MD, Myers TJ, Frazier OH, Cooley DA. Thirty-five years of mechanical circulatory support at the Texas Heart Institute: an updated overview. Tex Heart Inst J 2005;32:168–77.

[11] Song X, Throckmorton AL, Untaroiu A, Patel S, Allaire PE, Wood HG, Olsen DB. Axial flow blood pumps. ASAIO J 2003;49:355–64.

[12] Noon GP, Lafuente JA, Irwin S. Acute and temporary ventricular support with Bio-Medicus centrifugal pump. Ann ThoracSurg 1999;68:650–4.

[13] Vranckx P, Foley DP, de Feijter PJ, Vos J, Smits P, Serruys PW. Clinical introduction of the Tandemheart, a percutaneous left ventricular assist device, for circulatory support during high-risk percutaneous coronary intervention. Int J CardiovascIntervent 2003;5:35–9.

http://dx.doi.org/10.5772/55918

[14] Scalia GM, McCarthy PM, Savage RM, Smedira NG, Thomas JD. Clinical utility of echocardiography in the management of implantable ventricular assist devices. J Am SocEchocardiogr 2000;13:754–63.

[15] Myers TJ, Robertson K, Pool T, Shah N, Gregoric I, Frazier OH. Continuous flow pumps and total artificial hearts: management issues. Ann ThoracSurg 2003;75: S79-85.

[16] Myers TJ, Bolmers M, Gregoric ID, Kar B, Frazier OH. Assessment of arterial blood pressure during support with an axial flow left ventricular assist device.J Heart Lung Transplant 2009 May;28(5):423-7.

[17] Vitarelli A, Gheorghiade M. Transthoracic and transesophageal echocardiography in the hemodynamic assessment of patients with congestive heart failure. Am J Cardiol 2000; 86:36–40.

[18] Nussmeier NA, Probert CB, Hirsch D, Cooper JR Jr, Gregoric ID, Myers TJ, Frazier OH. Anesthetic management for implantation of the Jarvik 2000 left ventricular assist system. AnesthAnalg 2003;97:964–71.

[19] Rao V, Slater JP, Edwards NM, Naka Y, Oz MC. Surgical management of valvular disease in patients requiring left ventricular assist device support. Ann ThoracSurg 2001;71:1448–53.

[20] Holman WL, Bourge RC, Fan P, Kirklin JK, Pacifico AD, Nanda NC. Influence of left ventricular assist on valvular regurgitation. Circulation 1993;88:309–18.

[21] Gruber EM, Seitelberger R, Mares P, Hiesmayr MJ. Ventricular thrombus and subarachnoid bleeding during support with ventricular assist devices. Ann ThoracSurg 1999;67:1778–80.

[22] Lacroix V, d'Udekem Y, Jacquet L, Noirhomme P. Resection of the ascending aorta and aortic valve patch closure for type A aortic dissection after Novacor LVAD insertion. Eur J CardiothoracSurg 2003;24:309–11.

[23] Momeni M, Van Caenegem O, Van DyckMJ.Aortic regurgitation after left ventricular assist device placement. J CardiothoracVascAnesth 2005;19:409–10.

[24] Bryant AS, Holman WL, Nanda NC, Vengala S, Blood MS, Pamboukian SV, Kirklin JK. Native aortic valve insufficiency in patients with left ventricular assist devices. Ann ThoracSurg 2006;81:E6–8.

[25] Pelletier MP, Chang CP, Vagelos R, Robbins RC.Alternative approach for use of a left ventricular assist device with a thrombosed prosthetic valve. J Heart Lung Transplant 2002;21:402–4.

[26] Connelly JH, Abrams J, Klima T, Vaughn WK, Frazier OH. Acquired commissural fusion of aortic valves in patients with left ventricular assist devices. J Heart Lung Transplant 2003;22:1291–5.

[27] Rose AG, Connelly JH, Park SJ, Frazier OH, Miller LW, Ormaza S. Total left ventricular outflow tract obstruction due to left ventricular assist device-induced sub-aortic thrombosis in 2 patients with aortic valve bioprosthesis. J Heart Lung Transplant 2003;22:594–9.

[28] Koelling TM, Aaronson KD, Cody RJ, Bach DS, Armstrong WF. Prognostic significance of mitral regurgitation and tricuspid regurgitation in patients with left ventricular systolic dysfunction. Am Heart J 2002;144:524–9.

[29] Gibson TC, Foale RA, Guyer DE, Weyman AE. Clinical significance of incomplete tricuspid valve closure seen on two-dimensional echocardiography. J Am CollCardiol 1984;4:1052–7.

[30] Bursi F, Enriquez-Sarano M, Nkomo VT, Jacobsen SJ, Weston SA, Meverden RA, Roger VL. Heart failure and death after myocardial infarction in the community: the emerging role of mitral regurgitation. Circulation 2005;111:295–301.

[31] Schmid C, Radovancevic B. When should we consider right ventricular support? J ThoracCardiovascSurg 2002;50:204–7.

[32] Santamore WP, Gray LA Jr. Left ventricular contributions to right ventricular systolic function during LVAD support. Ann ThoracSurg 1996;61:350–6.

[33] Kawai A, Kormos RL, Mandarino WA, Morita S, Deneault LG, Gasior TA, Armitage JM, Griffith BP. Differential regional function of the right ventricle during the use of a left ventricular assist device. ASAIO J 1992;38:M676–8.

[34] Miller LW. Patient selection for the use of ventricular assist devices as a bridge to transplantation. Ann ThoracSurg2003;75:S66–71.

[35] Ochiai Y, McCarthy PM, Smedira NG, Banbury MK, Navia JL, Feng J, Hsu AP, Yeager ML, Buda T, Hoercher KJ, Howard MW, Takagaki M, Doi K, Fukamachi K. Predictors of severe right ventricular failure after implantable left ventricular assist device insertion: analysis of 245 patients. Circulation 2002;106:I198–202.

[36] Fukamachi K, McCarthy PM, Smedira NG, Vargo RL, Starling RC, Young JB. Preoperative risk factors for right ventricular failure after implantable left ventricular assist device insertion. Ann ThoracSurg 1999;68:2181–4.

[37] Mendes LA, Picard MH, Sleeper LA, Thompson CR, Jacobs AK, White HD, Hochman JS, Davidoff R. Cardiogenic shock: predictors of outcome based on right and left ventricular size and function at presentation. Coron Artery Dis 2005;16:209–15.

[38] Maslow AD, Regan MM, Panzica P, Heindel S, Mashikian J, Comunale ME. Pre-cardiopulmonary bypass right ventricular function is associated with poor outcome after coronary artery bypass grafting in patients with severe left ventricular systolic dysfunction. AnesthAnalg 2002;95:1507–18.

[39] Vaur L, Abergel E, Laaban JP, Raffoul H, Jeanrenaud X, Diebold B. Quantitative analysis of systolic function of the right ventricule by Doppler echocardiography. Arch Mal Coeur Vaiss 1991;84:89–93.

[40] Yamada S, Nakatani S, Imanishi T, Nakasone I, Sunagawa K, Miyatake K. Estimation of right ventricular contractility by continuous-wave Doppler echocardiography. J Cardiol 1996; 28:287–93.

[41] Stainback RF, Croitoru M, Hernandez A, Myers TJ, Wadia Y, Frazier OH. Echocardiographic evaluation of the Jarvik 2000 axial-flow LVAD. Tex Heart Inst J 2005;32(3):263-70.

[42] Sun BC, Catanese KA, Spanier TB, Flannery MR, Gardocki MT, Marcus LS, Levin HR, Rose EA, Oz MC. 100 long-term implantable left ventricular assist devices: the Columbia Presbyterian interim experience. Ann ThoracSurg 1999;68:688–94.

[43] Dandel M, Weng Y, Siniawski H, Potapov E, Lehmkuhl HB, Hetzer R. Long-term results in patients with idiopathic dilated cardiomyopathy after weaning from left ventricular assist devices. Circulation 2005;112:I37–45.

[44] Slaughter MS, Silver MA, Farrar DJ, Tatooles AJ, Pappas PS. A new method of monitoring recovery and weaning the Thoratec left ventricular assist device. Ann ThoracSurg 2001;71:215–18.

[45] Hetzer R, Muller JH, Weng Y, Meyer R, Dandel M. Bridging-to-recovery. Ann ThoracSurg 2001;71:S109–13; discussion S114–15.

[46] Khan T, Delgado RM, Radovancevic B, Torre-Amione G, Abrams J, Miller K, Myers T, Okerberg K, Stetson SJ, Gregoric I, Hernandez A, Frazier OH. Dobutamine stress echocardiography predicts myocardial improvement in patients supported by left ventricular assist devices (LVADs): hemodynamic and histologic evidence of improvement before LVAD explantation. J Heart Lung Transplant 2003;22:137–46.

[47] Chen JM, Levin HR, Rose EA, Addonizio LJ, Landry DW, Sistino JJ, Michler RE, Oz MC. Experience with right ventricular assist devices for perioperative right-sided circulatory failure. Ann ThoracSurg 1996;61:305–10; discussion 311–13.

[48] Vincent JL, Rhodes A, Perel A, Martin GS, Della Rocca G, Vallet B, Pinsky MR, Hofer CK, Teboul JL, de Boode WP, Scolletta S, Vieillard-Baron A, De Backer D, Walley KR, Maggiorini M, Singer M. Clinical review: Update on hemodynamic monitoring-a consensus of 16. Crit Care 2011; 18;15(4):229.

[49] Tsutsui M, Matsuoka N, Ikeda T, Sanjo Y, Kazama T. Comparison of a new cardiac output ultrasound dilution method with thermodilution technique in adult patients under general anesthesia. J CardiothoracVascAnesth 2009; 23:835–840.

[50] Scolletta S, Miraldi F, Romano SM, Muzzi L. Continuous cardiac output monitoring with an uncalibrated pulse contour method in patients supported with mechanical pulsatile assist device. Interact CardioVascThoracSurg 2011;13:52–57.

[51] Shah MR, Hasselblad V, Stevenson LW, Binanay C, O'Connor CM, Sopko G, Califf RM. Impact of the pulmonary artery catheter in critically ill patients: meta-analysis of randomized clinical trials. JAMA 2005;294:1664–1670.

[52] Schmid ER, Schmidlin D, Tornic M, Seifert B. Continuous thermodilution cardiac output: clinical validation against a reference technique of known accuracy. Intensive Care Med 1999;25(2):166–72.

[53] Goedje O, Hoeke K, Lichtwarck-Aschoff M, Faltchauser A, Lamm P, Reichart B. Continuous cardiac output by femoral arterial thermodilution calibrated pulse contour analysis: comparison with pulmonary arterial thermodilution. Crit Care Med 1999;27:2407–2412.

[54] Gondos T, Marjanek Z, Kisvarga Z, Halász G. Precision of transpulmonary thermodilution: how many measurements are necessary? Eur J Anaesthesiol 2009;26(6):508–12.

[55] Linton NWF, Linton RAF. Estimation of changes in cardiac output from the arterial blood pressure waveform in the upper limb. Br J Anaesth 2001;86:486–96.

[56] Mets B, Frumento RJ, Bennett-Guerrero E, Naka Y. Validation of continuous thermodilution cardiac output in patients implanted with a left ventricular assist device. J CardiothoracVascAnesth 2002;16:727–730.

[57] Thiele RH, Durieux ME. Arterial waveform analysis for the anesthesiologist: past, present, and future concepts. AnesthAnalg2011;113:766-776.

[58] Wesseling KH, Jansen JRC, Settels JJ, Schreuder JJ. Computation of aortic flow pressure in humans using a nonlinear, threeelement model. J ApplPhysiol 1993;74: 2566–73.

[59] Giraud R, Siegenthaler N, Bendjelid K. Transpulmonary thermodilution assessments: precise measurements require a precise procedure.Crit Care 2011;15(5):195.

[60] Cecconi M, Dawson D, Grounds RM, Rhodes A. Lithium dilution cardiac output measurement in the critically ill patient: determination of precision of the technique. Intensive Care Med 2009;35(3):498–504.

[61] Monnet X, Anguel N, Jozwiak M, Richard C, Teboul JL. Third-generation FloTrac/Vigileo does not reliably track changes in cardiac output induced by norepinephrine in critically ill patients. Br J Anaesth 2012;108(4):615–22.

[62] Scolletta S, Franchi F, Taccone FS, Donadello K, Biagioli B, Vincent JL.An uncalibrated pulse contour method to measure cardiac output during aortic counterpulsation. AnesthAnalg 2011;113(6):1389-95.

[63] Scolletta S, Muzzi L, Romano SM, Gregoric ID, Frazier HO. The "left" ventricle during pulsatile mechanical assistance: reliability of cardiac output monitoring with an uncalibrated pulse contour method. Eur Heart J 2010;31(2):148.

[64] Wiesenack C, Prasser C, Liebold A, Schmid FX. Assessment of left ventricular cardiac output by arterial thermodilution technique via a left atrial catheter in a patient on a right ventricular assist device. Perfusion 2004;19:73–75.

[65] Riha H, Kotulak T, Syrovatka P, Netuka I. Hemodynamic monitoring with LiDCO-plus system in the patients supported by isolated right ventricular assist device. Interact CardiovascThoracSurg 2011;13(1):57.

[66] Scolletta S, Gregoric ID, Muzzi L, Radovancevic B, Frazier OH. Pulse wave analysis to assess systemic blood flow during mechanical biventricular support. Perfusion 2007;22(1):63–6.

[67] Frazier OH, Myers TJ, Westaby S, Gregoric ID. Clinical experience with an implantable, intracardiac, continuous flow circulatory support device: physiologic implications and their relationship to patient selection. Ann ThoracSurg 2004;77:133–42.

[68] Romano SM, Pistolesi M. Assessment of cardiac output from systemic arterial pressure in humans. Crit Care Med 2002;30:1834–1841.

[69] Montenij LJ, de Waal EE, Buhre WF. Arterial waveform analysis in anesthesia and critical care.CurrOpinAnaesthesiol 2011;24(6):651–6.

[70] Camporota L, Beale R. Pitfalls in haemodynamic monitoring based on the arterial pressure waveform. Crit Care 2010;14:124.

Section 2

Major Complications and Future Prospects of Ventricular Assist Devices

Chapter 3

Gastrointestinal Bleeding with Continuous Flow Left Ventricular Assist Devices (LVADs)

Geetha Bhat, Mukesh Gopalakrishnan and Ashim Aggarwal

Additional information is available at the end of the chapter

http://dx.doi.org/10.5772/56010

1. Introduction

Continuous flow left ventricular assist devices (CF-LVADs) have emerged as the standard of care for patients in advanced heart failure. The two common CF-LVADs in use are the FDA approved HeartMate II® (Thoratec Inc.) and the currently investigational HVAD™ (HeartWare Inc.). These CF-LVADs are being used as a bridge-to-transplant (BTT) and also as destination therapy (DT) (for those ineligible for heart transplant) [1, 2]. The clinical use of these newer devices has resulted in improved outcomes [3] including significantly reduced complication rates with improved durability compared to the first generation pulsatile design pumps [2]. However, with this new technology, a new set of complications have arisen including the increased incidence of Gastrointestinal (GI) bleeding [4, 5, 6, 7].

2. Definition

Patients are considered to have GI bleeding if they have one or more of the following symptoms: guaiac-positive stools, hematemesis, hematochezia, melena, active bleeding or blood within the GI tract at the time of endoscopy or colonoscopy, drop in hematocrit or patients hemoglobin level decreases by more than or equal to 1g/dl which necessitates transfusion of packed red blood cells [4, 5]

3. Incidence

Several studies done on CF-LVADs have shown varying rates of GI bleed ranging from 15% to 50% [Table 1]. One series showed that CF-LVADs have nearly four times the incidence of bleeding compared to the pulsatile devices [8].

Author	Study Population	Device	BTT / DT	GI Bleed Incidence	Results
Letsou et al. J Heart Lung Transplant 2005;24:105-109 [9]	21	JARVIK 2000	21 / -	3 (14%)	• All three cases were secondary to AVMs in the GI tract.
Stern et al. J Card Surg 2010;25:352-356 [7]	33	HM II® (20)/ HM XVE® (9)/ VentrAssist® (4)	19 / 14	8 out of 20 HM II® patients (40%)	• GI bleed was noticed only in patients with HM II® LVAD. • 3 patients (38%) had rebleeds • Mean time to first GI bleed was 87 days. • Source of bleed was identifiable in only 6(35%) patients.
Uriel et al. J Am Coll Caridol 2010;56:1207-12 13 [10]	79	HM II®	64 / 15	24 (30.3%)	• Aim of the study was looking at bleeding from all cause. • GI bleed analysis was secondary.
Demirozu et al. J Heart Lung Transplant 2011;30:849-53 [5]	172	HM II®	-	32 (19%)	• AVMs were source of bleeding in 10 (32%) patients. • Median time to first GI bleed was 40 days. • All 4 patients with a previous history of GI bleed, bled again.
John et al. Ann Thorac Surg 2011;92:1593-16 00 [11]	130	HM II®	102 / -	18 (17.6%)	• Analysis of GI bleed was not the primary end point of the study.
Morgan et al.	86	HM II®	54 / 32	19 (22.1%)	• Previous history of GI bleed was an independent

Author	Study Population	Device	BTT / DT	GI Bleed Incidence	Results
J Heart Lung Transplant 2012;31:715-718 [6]					predictor of future GI bleeds (OR 2.24). • Patients with previous history of GI bleed, bled more (p=0.01) • All recurrent bleeds were from the same site.
Aggarwal et al. Ann Thorac Surg 2012;93:1534-1540 [4]	101	HM II®	7 / 94	23 (22.8%)	• Previous history of GI bleeds (OR 22.7), elevated INR (OR 3.9) and low platelets (OR -0.98) were independent predictors of future GI bleeds. • Most common cause of bleeding was gastric erosions followed by AVMs. • Recurrent bleed was more common in elderly patients. • Octreotide did not impact clinical outcomes.

GI – Gastrointestinal; AVM – Arteriovenous Malformation; HM II® – HeartMate II®; HM XVE – HeartMate XVE®; BTT – Bridge to Transplant; DT – Destination Therapy; INR – International Normalized Ratio; HMW vWF – High Molecular, LVAD- Left ventricular assist device, Weight vonWillebrand Factor; OR – Odds Ratio

Table 1. Studies evaluating GI bleed in LVAD patients

4. Pathophysiology

The first generation of LVADs (HeartMate I®) utilized a pulsatile flow mechanism that did not necessitate anticoagulation like the newer second generation pumps. Reports of GI bleeding do however exist with this device [12, 13]. Since the advent of the newer CF-LVADs, the incidence of GI bleed has increased. Multiple mechanisms for this have been proposed: coagulopathy, lack of pulsatility, acquired vonWillebrand syndrome (AvWS) or other risk factors (low platelet count, increased age and a previous history of GI bleed) (Fig. 1.).

Patients with CF-LVADs have state physiologically similar to aortic stenosis because of the narrow pulse pressure [4, 14]. Heyde et al. [15, 16] suggested this physiology resulting in distension of the sub-mucosal venous plexus of GI tract eventually leading to angiodysplasia, arteriovenous malformations (AVMs) and bleeding. An alternative mechanism that has been suggested describes decreased perfusion of the GI and intestinal mucosa due to low pulse pressure, causing mucosal ischemia and the formation of friable new vessels that are likely to bleed [5]. Several other theories have also been proposed for the relation between aortic stenosis like flow pattern and GI bleeding. Boley and colleagues [17] suggested that increased intraluminal pressure with muscular contraction may result in dilated mucosal veins that favor development of AV communication which may bleed when exposed to trauma or stress. Alternatively a neurovascular cause proposed by Cappell and colleagues [18] indicates that increased sympathetic tone results in smooth muscle relaxation and development of angiodysplasia.

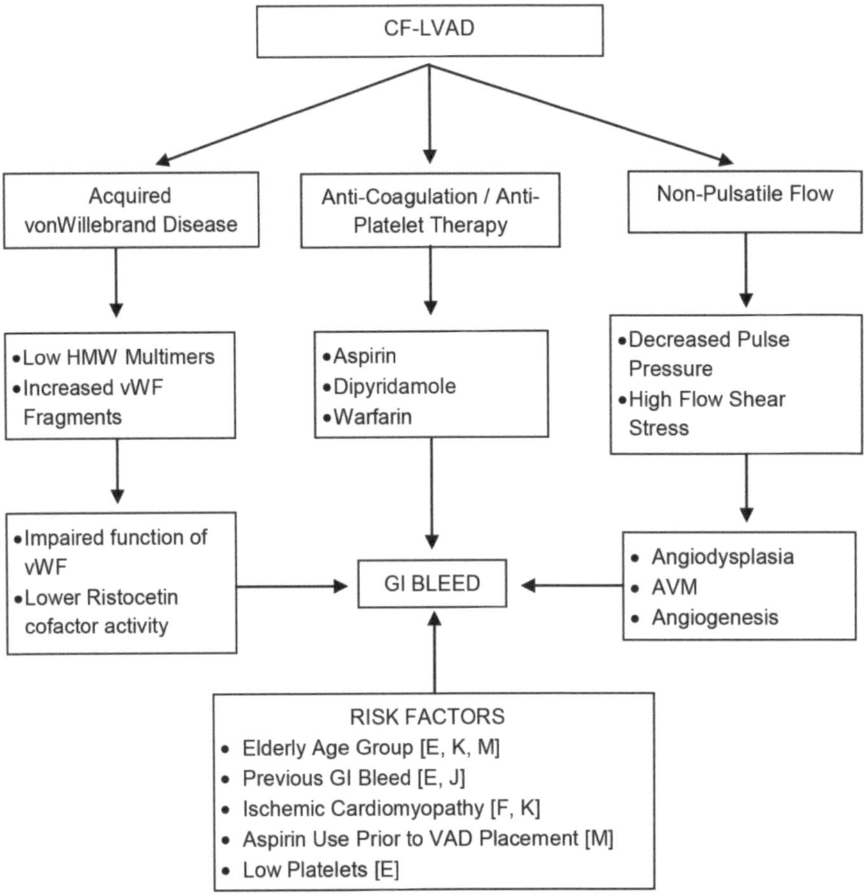

HMW – High Molecular Weight; vWF – VonWillebrand Factor; AVM – ArterioVenous Malformation

Figure 1. Pathophysiology of GI bleeding in CF-LVAD

There is a substantial alteration of the prothrombotic profile in patients with CF-LVADs. The integrity of vascular endothelium, as evidenced by border protein expressions such as vonWillebrand Factor (vWF), is partially dependent on the stretch and distension created by the pulsatile flow. This plays an important homeostatic role in areas of high sheer stress such as GI AVMs [19, 20, 21]. One mechanism that was initially noted by Uriel et al. [10] was the development of AvWS as supported by depletion of high molecular weight vWF. CF-LVADs have impellar-like mechanism which creates high sheer stress environment and causes elongation and unfolding of the vWF multimers resulting in exposure to metalloproteases that cleaves it to form smaller vWF multimers similar to what happens when blood flows across a stenotic aortic valve [22, 23]. Sixty percent of patients with low HMW vWF experienced bleeding. Klovaite et al. [19] demonstrated the impact of CF-LVAD on vWF dependent platelet aggregation. They showed that almost 70% of the patients had impaired ristocetin-induced platelet aggregation. These labs return to normal baseline values post heart transplant which suggests that the hemodynamics of CF-LVADs have a significant role to play [10, 14].

5. Contributing factors

Major bleeding events are seen more frequently in older population and in those with ischemic cardiomyopathy as their underlying etiology for heart failure [10] (Fig. 1.). One of the most significant contributing factors is a previous history of GI bleed with the most likely source of bleed being the same site as the previous bleed [4]. Those with multiple episodes of bleeding tend to be significantly older than those with a single episode of bleed [4]. These patients need to be evaluated carefully preceding LVAD implantation because of their elevated risk profile. The duration of LVAD implantation does not appear to play a significant role as bleeding occurs at varying time intervals ranging from 8 to 18 months. Recent study by Aggarwal et al. [4] showed that an INR value at the upper limit of goal increased the risk of GI bleed compared to the lower limit, although this was not statistically significant. Platelets counts were also significantly lower in those with GI bleed according to the same study [4].

6. Classification of GI bleed

Bleeding is classified as either upper GI (proximal to the ligament of Treitz, which includes the esophagus, stomach and duodenum) or lower GI (distal to the ligament of Treitz, which includes the jejunum, ileum and colon) based on the site of bleed. Most common causes are vascular malformations like AVM and Dieulafoy lesions accounting for 30 - 40% and 15 - 20% respectively and peptic ulcer disease accounting for 10 - 15%. The location and types of lesions causing GI bleed are listed in Table 2 as seen from 4 different studies on this topic [4, 5, 7, 24].

7. Management

Management of a LVAD patient with GI bleed utilizes a multi-disciplinary approach. Main goals of initial assessment should be to evaluate the location and severity of bleed, hold any anti-coagulants and resuscitate to maintain stable hemodynamics (Fig. 2.).

Upper GI
Gastric / Duodenal AVM
Gastric / Duodenal Dieulafoy Lesions
Hemorrhagic Gastritis
Esophageal / Gastric / Duodenal Ulcers
Gastric Polyps
Gastric Angiodysplasia
Mallory Weiss Tear
Cameron's Ulcers
Lower GI
Jejunal / Colonic AVMs
Small Bowel Angiodysplasia
Diverticulosis
Cecal / Rectal Ulcers
Ischemic Colitis
Sigmoid Polyp
Hemorrhoids
Drive-Line Erosions of the Colon

Table 2. Location of GI bleeding after CF-LVAD

7.1. Laboratory investigations

Blood counts with hemoglobin and hematocrit along with platelet count need to be evaluated and compared with patient's most recent baseline value to assess severity of the bleed. Bleeding profile of the patient should also be obtained to assess level of coagulopathy.

7.2. Blood products

These include transfusion of packed red blood cells, platelets, cryoprecipitate and fresh frozen plasma as clinically indicated. The latter is usually given if there is evidence of active bleeding especially with supratherapeutic PT/INR. Transfusion requirements averaged 2 - 4 units of packed red blood cell per bleeding patient as shown in multiple studies [4, 5, 7].

7.3. Pharmacotherapy

7.3.1. Anticoagulants / antiplatelets

The current standard of treatment involves immediate discontinuation of antiplatelets and anticoagulants including aspirin, dipyridamole and warfarin. Although discontinuation of anticoagulants poses a risk for development of device thrombosis and subsequent systemic embolus, the true incidence of this adverse event is low. This has been attributed to be sintered titanium lining the inner surface of these devices [20, 25]. There are cases that have reported discontinuation of anticoagulants (in recurrent GI bleeders) for prolonged periods (up to 12 months) without any incidence of thrombus formation [26]. Anticoagulants are temporarily withheld and are restarted after complete resolution of bleeding. Patients with previous history or at high risk of thrombosis might require bridging (till INR reaches therapeutic range) with unfractionated or low molecular weight heparin, while being closely monitored for signs of bleeding.

7.3.2. *Proton Pump Inhibitors (PPI)*

High dose antisecretory therapy with proton pump inhibitors like omeprazole, pantoprazole significantly reduce the rate of bleeding and rebleeding from GI ulcers [27]. PPI therapy also promotes hemostasis in lesions other than ulcers by neutralizing gastric acid which leads to stabilization of the clots [28]. Oral and intravenous PPI therapy also decreases rebleeding rate, the length of hospital stay and need for blood transfusion in patients [29, 30].

7.3.3. *Octreotide*

This is a synthetic somatostatin analogue that is usually used in the treatment of variceal bleeding but has been shown to reduce the risk of bleeding due to non-variceal causes as well [31]. It has been used in some centers with mixed reports. It acts by inhibiting gastric acid, decreasing gut hormones as well as constricting splanchnic and portal circulation. It also inhibits growth factors such as endothelial growth factors, basic fibroblast growth factor, and insulin-like growth factor-1 and is responsible for suppression of angiogenesis [32]. It can be administered either as a continuous infusion or subcutaneous injection [33]. Aggarwal and colleagues [4] demonstrated that octreotide administration did not significantly impact the length of hospital stay, requirements for blood transfusion, rebleeding rates or mortality. However these results could have been skewed because the predominant cause of the GI bleeding in their study population was gastric erosions with AVMs a close second.

7.4. Diagnostic modalities

There are multiple diagnostic modalities available to investigate and visualize the source of GI bleed. However, the source of bleed might not be identifiable in all cases. One study reported the possibility of not being able to locate the site of bleed at 65% of their study population [24].

7.4.1. *Esophagogastroduodenoscopy (EGD)*

This allows direct visualization of the esophagus, stomach and the proximal duodenum. EGD also permits us to perform intervention if needed at a site of bleeding which could be an AVM or Dieulafoy lesion. Elmunzer et al. [24] demonstrated that on average 3.3 endoscopic procedures were necessary for each patient before the cause of bleeding was established and several require an additional procedure prior to achieving complete hemostasis. Complications for this procedure include bowel perforation, bleeding, aspiration pneumonia and complication related to sedation.

7.4.2. *Colonoscopy*

This procedure provides us with direct visualization of the mucosa of the cecum, colon and rectum. Advantages include its ability to localize the site of bleed and the potential for interventional therapy. Some gastroenterologists do not recommend any bowel preparation since blood is a cathartic while others prefer an enema or a quick bowel preparation with balanced electrolyte solution [34]. The cecum can be reached in 95 % of patients presenting with lower GI bleed which may be sufficient enough as most lesions are found distal to the cecum [34]. Complications of this procedure include bowel perforation, bleeding, infection and complications secondary to sedation.

7.4.3. Small bowel Video Capsule Endoscopy (VCE)

This provides a non-invasive diagnostic imaging of the small intestine that cannot be visualized with an EGD. The overall yield for obscure GI bleeding has been reported to be in the range of 45 – 70% with one meta-analysis showing the diagnostic yield of VCE (63%) to be significantly higher than deep bowel enteroscopy (26%) [35]. In about 16% of cases it does not reach the cecum within the recording time due to various reasons that can cause the bowel motility to slow down [36]. The main disadvantage with this study is that it is not possible to intervene therapeutically. There is some concern that the wireless signal transmission from capsule may be disturbed by the electromagnetic field of the VAD. The opposite may also be of concern where the signals may interfere with the functioning of the VAD and ICD [37, 38]. However, patients have undergone these procedures without complications.

7.4.4. Tagged RBC bleeding scan

Radionuclide imaging study can detect blood loss occurring at a rate of 0.1 – 0.5 ml/min. It is more sensitive than angiography but less specific [44]. The major disadvantage is that this can only localize the bleed to a general area in the abdomen and not a precise location. Tagged RBC scan should typically be performed prior to angiography to determine if bleeding is sufficient enough to increase the diagnostic yield of an angiogram and allow for selective angiography of appropriate vessels. Patients with a negative bleeding scan are most likely to have a negative angiogram [45].

7.4.5. Mesenteric angiogram

Angiography requires active blood loss of 1 – 1.5 ml/min for a bleeding site to be visualized [42]. This procedure is very specific but sensitivity varies depending on the pattern of bleeding. Advantages with this procedure are accurate anatomic localization of bleed and the fact that it does not need any bowel preparation. It permits therapeutic intervention with catheter directed vasopressin infusion and transcatheter embolization. The frequency of a negative arteriogram can be reduced if radionuclide imaging is used to screen for active bleeding [43]. Disadvantages include the inability to use this with renal insufficiency. Complications include worsening of renal function, infarction, bleeding.

7.4.6. Deep bowel enteroscopy

Deep small bowel enteroscopy permits visualization and intervention till upto 60 cm of the proximal jejunum. The procedure is approached from the mouth (anterograde) or from the anus (retrograde) depending on whether the lesion is found in the first 60 % of VCE or in the last 40 % [39]. The diagnostic yield of balloon assisted enteroscopy ranges from 40 – 80 % with therapy being performed in 20 – 55 % of patients [40, 41]. Complications of this procedure include pancreatitis, bowel perforation, bleeding, and aspiration pneumonia.

7.5. Device management

The usual speeds of a LVAD pump are maintained at 8800 – 10000 rpm (for axial flow HM II®) and 2800 – 3200 rpm (for centrifugal flow HVAD™). In a patient with GI bleed, a common practice is to reduce the VAD pump speed to generate pulsatility. Speed adjustment should ideally be performed under echocardiographic monitoring in order to achieve the lowest possible speed safely while ensuring adequate left ventricular unloading [4]. This however might not be possible at time in patients with severe bleeding

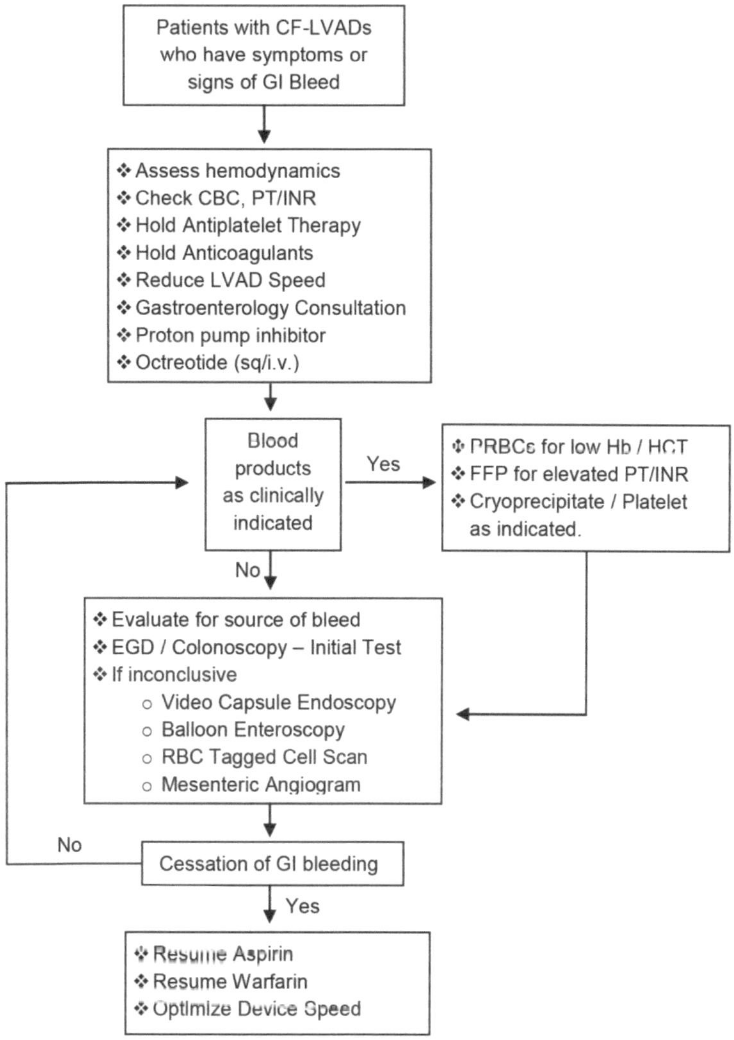

CBC – Complete Blood Count; PT – Prothrombin Time; sq - Subcutaneous ; i.v. Intravenous; Hb - Hemoglobin; HCT-Hematocrit; EGD – Esophagogastroduodenoscopy; PRBC – Packed Red Blood Cell

Figure 2. Management of GI bleeds in CF-LVADs

7.6. Intervention

Endoscopic interventional technique includes cauterization, injection, and clipping of a visible vessel, while intervention with mesenteric angiography involves transcatheter coil embolization. It is possible to perform a Deep Bowel Push Enteroscopy as a diagnostic and therapeutic procedure potentially guided by results of the capsule endoscopy. This is a somewhat invasive procedure but a good alternative to the more invasive surgical laparotomy. Very rarely surgical procedures like partial gastrectomy or bowel resection are required after multiple failed attempts at other non-surgical treatment options.

7.7. Anticoagulation post GI bleed

Aspirin is usually restarted after cessation of GI bleeding and ensuring hemodynamic stability. Re-initiation of warfarin along with aspirin is variable and depends on the severity of the GI bleed, endoscopic appearance of culprit lesion and other comorbidities (e.g. prosthetic heart valve). Goal INR for those anticoagulated with warfarin post GI bleed is aimed at the lower end of the therapeutic range (1.5 – 2 for HM II® and 2 – 3 for HVAD™) [4, 46].

7.8. Recurrence of GI bleed

Recurrence is more common in patients restarted on warfarin in combination with aspirin compared to those on aspirin alone. It is more common in the elderly and almost 60% of these recurrences are from the same site of bleed as the original source [4]. The predominant cause is usually gastric angiodysplasia [7]. After resuscitation and management of the bleed, the practice of restarting anticoagulation with warfarin varies widely and depends on patient comorbidities and physician preference. If it is restarted, goal INR is usually maintained close to lower end of normal for the specific LVAD type [4, 46]. Few preventive strategies being promoted include (i) maintaining LVAD pump speed at the lowest possible safe range under echocardiographic guidance to reduce flow and gain relative pulsatility, (ii) maintain INR at the low end of the recommended range for the respective devices in patients at high risk of GI bleed, (iii) close outpatient monitoring (more frequent than usual outpatient monitoring) of INR, hemoglobin and platelets, (iv) having a low threshold for diagnostic endoscopic evaluation in patients suspected of having GI bleeding.

8. Future directions

The significance of the role played by anticoagulants in causing GI bleeding along with altered hemodynamics and AvWS is not clearly discernable. Patient specific anticoagulation may be required tom improve clinical outcomes. Studies have shown that genetic polymorphisms in cytochrome P450 2C9 (CYP2C9) and vitamin K epoxide reductase gene (VKORC1) affect the pharmacokinetics and pharmacodynamics of warfarin [47]. Warfarin genotyping has been proven to reduce hospitalization rates including those due to GI bleeding [48] but has not been evaluated in this particular population with CF-LVADs.

The use of direct thrombin inhibitors like dabigatran, and Factor Xa inhibitors like apixaban and rivaroxaban has been approved for stroke prophylaxis in non-valvular atrial fibrillation [49, 50,

http://dx.doi.org/10.5772/56010

51]. No studies have been done testing the efficacy of these newer anticoagulants in patient with CF-LVADs. Future trials could be directed towards this to look for suitable alternatives to warfarin.

The use of thalidomide for GI bleeding secondary to vascular malformation that is refractory to endoscopic or medical therapy has been mentioned in literature. Thalidomide has anti-inflammatory, immunomodulatory and anti-angiogenic properties along with the capability to inhibit vascular endothelial growth factor (VEGF), a key component in the formation of vascular endothelium in the early stages of angiogenesis [52]. In a study by Ge et al. [53], it has shown to be an effective and safe method for treating and preventing recurrent GI bleeding for a period of up to 1 year. Lenalidomide, a thalidomide analogue that is more potent with lesser side effects is being evaluated for the same. There have not been any case reports regarding the use of thalidomide or its analogue in GI bleeding with CF-LVADs.

Another new avenue for treatment of GI bleed in LVAD patients involves the possible use of Factor VIII concentrates that contain both Factor VIII and vWF (Haemate P / Humate-P) for AvWS. Cushing et al. [54] reported a single case where transfusion of Factor VIII resulted in a significant decrease in the requirement for blood component transfusion. Once the treatment was initiated, the levels of vWF activity and Factor VIII levels improved dramatically. Future studies could investigate this possibility as a novel therapeutic strategy.

The likelihood of establishing pulsatile flow, even if intermittently with CF-LVADs has to be entertained in the future. If change in hemodynamics with continuous flow rather than pulsatile flow is a major contributor for GI bleeding then this might help reduce the number of events in the future. Newer devices may have this capability built in to switch back and forth between the two pump modes.

9. Conclusion

GI bleeding from CF-LVADs is gaining prominence with increasing use of CF-LVADs as a BTT or DT in those with refractory heart failure. At the present time there is no clear evidence that indicates a distinctive way in which to treat all GI bleeds. Management strategy depends on the patient's clinical picture, aggressive supportive measures and timely intervention.

Author details

Geetha Bhat[1*], Mukesh Gopalakrishnan[2] and Ashim Aggarwal[1]

*Address all correspondence to: geetha.bhat@advocatehealth.com

1 Center for Heart Transplant and Assist Devices, Advocate Christ Medical Center, Oak Lawn, USA

2 Department of Internal Medicine, Advocate Illinois Masonic Medical Center, Chicago, USA

References

[1] Miller LW. Use of a Continuous-Flow Device in Patients Awaiting Heart Transplantation. N Eng J Med 2007; 357:885-89

[2] Slaughter MS. Advanced Heart Failure treated with continuous-flow left ventricular assist devices: N Eng J Med 2009;361:2241-51

[3] John R. Improved Survival and Decreasing Incidence of Adverse Events with the HeartMate II Left Ventricular Assist Device as Bridge-to-Transplant Therapy: Ann Thorac Surg 2009;86:1227-1235

[4] Aggarwal A. Incidence and Management of Gastrointestinal Bleeding With Continuous Flow Assist Devices: Ann Thoracic Surg 2012;93:1534-40

[5] Demirozu ZT. Arteriovenous malformations and gastrointestinal bleeding in patients with HeartMate II left ventricular assist device: J Heart Lung Transplant 2011;30:849-53

[6] Morgan JA. Gastrointestinal bleeding with the HeartMate II left ventricular assist device: J Heart Lung Transplant 2012;31:715-718

[7] Stern DR. Increased incidence of gastrointestinal bleeding following implantation of the HeartMate II LVAD: J Card Surg 2012;25:352-6

[8] Crow S. Gastrointestinal bleeding rates in recipients of nonpulsatile and pulsatile left ventricular assist devices: J Thorac Cardiovasc Surg 2009;137:208-15

[9] Lestou GV. GI Bleeding from Arterio-venous Malformations in Patients Supported by the Jarvik 2000 Axial Flow Left Ventricular Assist Device. J Heart Lung Transplant 2005;24:105-9

[10] Uriel N. Acquired von Willebrand syndrome after continuous-flow mechanical device support contributes to a high prevalence of bleeding during long-term support and at the time of transplantation: J Am Coll Cardiol 2012;56:1207-13

[11] John R. Lessons learned from experience with over 100 consecutive HeartMate II left ventricular assist devices: Ann Thorac Surg 2011;92:1593-9; discussion 1599-600

[12] McCarthy PM. One Hundred patients with HeartMate Left Ventricular Assist Device: Evolving Concepts and Technology. J Thorac Cardiovasc Surg 1998;115:904-912

[13] McBride. Clinical Experience with 111 Thoratec Ventricular Assist Devices. Ann Thorac Surg 1999;67:1233-1238

[14] Crow S. Acquired vonWillebrand Syndrome in Continuous-Flow Ventricular Assist Device Recipients: Ann Thorac Surg 2010;90:1263-1269

[15] Heyde EC. Gastrointestinal Bleeding in Aortic Stenosis. N Eng J Med 1958;259:196

[16] Islam S. Heyde's Syndrome: A critical review of the literature: J Heart Valve Dis 2011;20:366-75

[17] Boley SJ. On the nature and etiology of vascular ectasias of the colon. Degenerative lesions of aging. Gastroenterology 1977;72:650-60

[18] Cappell MS. Cessation of recurrent bleeding from gastrointestinal angiodysplasias after aortic valve replacement: Ann Intern Med 1986;105:54-7

[19] Klovaite J. Severely impaired von Willebrand's factor-dependent platelet aggregation in patients with a continuous –flow left ventricular assist device (HeartMate II): J Am Coll Cardiol 2009;53:2162-7

[20] John R. The biological basis of thrombosis and bleeding in patients with ventricular assist devices. J Cardiovasc Transl Res 2009;2:63-70

[21] Malehsa D. Acquired von Willebrand syndrome after exchange of the HeartMate XVE to the HeartMate II ventricular assist device: Eur J Cardiothorac Surg 2009;35:1091-3

[22] Baldauf C. Shear-induced Unfolding von Willberand Factor Activates A2 Doamin for Proteolysis. J Thromb Haemost 2009;7:2096-2105

[23] Warkentin TE. Aortic Stenosis and bleeding gastrointestinal angiodysplasia: is acquired von Willebrand's disease the link? Lancet 1992;340:35-7

[24] Elmunzer J. Endoscopic Findings and Clinical Outcomes in Ventricular Assist Device Recipients with Gastrointestinal Bleeding: Dig Dis Sci 2011;56:3241-3246

[25] Slaughter MS. Hematologic effects of continuous flow left ventricular assist devices: J Cardiovasc Transl Res 2010;3:618-24

[26] Pereira NL. Discontinuation of thrombotic therapy for a year or more in patients with continuous-flow left ventricular assist devices: Interact Cardiovasc Thorac Surg 2010; 11:503-5

[27] Chan WH. Randomized Control Trial of Standard versus High Dose Intravenous Omeprazole after Endoscopic Therapy in High-Risk Patients with Acute Peptic Ulcer Bleeding. Br J Surg. 2011;98(5):640

[28] Green FW Jr. Effect of acid and pepsin on blood coagulation and platelet aggregation. A possible contributor prolonged gastroduodenal mucosal hemorrhage. Gastroenterology. 1978;74(1):38

[29] Lee KK . Cost-effectiveness analysis of high-dose omeprazole infusion as adjuvant therapy to endoscopic treatment of bleeding peptic ulcer. Gastrointest Endosc. 2003;57(2):160

[30] Lau JY. Effect of intravenous omeprazole on recurrent bleeding after endoscopic treatment of bleeding peptic ulcers. N Engl J Med. 2000;343(5):310

[31] Imperiale TF. Somatostatin or octreotide compared with H2 antagonists and placebo in the management of acute nonvariceal upper gastrointestinal hemorrhage: a meta-analysis. Ann Intern Med. 1997;127(12):1062

[32] Blich M. Somatostatin therapy ameliorates chronic and refractory gastrointestinal bleeding caused by diffuse angiodysplasia in a patient on anticoagulation therapy: Scand J Gastroenterol 2003;38:801-3

[33] Nardone G. The efficacy of octreotide therapy in chronic bleeding due to vascular abnormalities of the gastrointestinal tract: Aliment Pharmacol Ther 1999;13:1429-36

[34] Rossini FP. Emergency colonoscopy. World J Surg. 1989;13(2):190

[35] Triester SL. A meta-analysis of the yield of capsule endoscopy compared to other diagnostic modalities in patients with obscure gastrointestinal bleeding. Am J Gastroenterol. 2005;100(11):2407

[36] Liao Z. Indications and detection, completion, and retention rates of small-bowel capsule endoscopy: a systematic review. Gastrointest Endosc. 2010;71(2):280

[37] Bechtel JFM. Localizing an occult gastrointestinal bleeding by wireless PillCam SB capsule video endoscopy in a patient with the HeartMate II left ventricular assist device: J Thorac Cardiovasc Surg 2010;139:e73-74

[38] Tarzia V. Occult gastrointestinal bleeding in patients with a left ventricular assist device axial flow pump; Diagnostic tools and therapeutic algorithm: J Thorac Cardiovasc Surg 2012;143:e28-31

[39] Li X. Predictive role of capsule endoscopy on the insertion route of double-balloon enteroscopy. Endoscopy. 2009;41(9):762

[40] Di Caro S. The European experience with double-balloon enteroscopy: indications, methodology, safety, and clinical impact. Gastrointest Endosc. 2005;62(4):545

[41] Gross SA. Initial experience with double-balloon enteroscopy at a U.S. center. Gastrointest Endosc. 2008;67(6):890

[42] Zuckerman DA. Massive hemorrhage in the lower gastrointestinal tract in adults: diagnostic imaging and intervention. AJR Am J Roentgenol. 1993;161(4):703

[43] Steer ML. Diagnostic procedures in gastrointestinal hemorrhage. N Engl J Med. 1983;309(11):646

[44] Dusold R. The accuracy of technetium-99m-labeled red cell scintigraphy in localizing gastrointestinal bleeding. Am J Gastroenterol. 1994;89(3):345

[45] Hunter JM. Limited value of technetium 99m-labeled red cell scintigraphy in localization of lower gastrointestinal bleeding. Am J Surg. 1990;159(5):504

[46] Slaughter MS. Clinical management of continuous-flow left ventricular assist devices in advance heart failure: J Heart Lung Transplant 2010;29(4 suppl):S1-39

http://dx.doi.org/10.5772/56010

[47] Shin J. Clinical Pharmacogenomics of Warfarin and Clopidogrel. Journal of Pharmacy Practice. http://jpp.sagepub.com/content/early/2012/05/10/0897190012448310

[48] Epstein RS. Warfarin Genotyping Reduces Hospitalization Rates. J Am Coll Cardiol 2010;55:2804–12)

[49] Connolly SJ. Dabigatran versus Warfarin in Patients with Atrial Fibrillation. N Eng J Med 2009;361:1139-1151

[50] Patel MR. Rivaroxaban versus Warfarin in Nonvalvular Atrial Fibrillation. N Eng J Med 2011;365:883-891

[51] Granger CB. Apixaban versus Warfarin in Patients with Atrial Fibrillation. N Eng J Med 2011;365:981-992

[52] Garrido A. Thalidomide in Refractory Bleeding due to Gastrointestinal Angiodysplasias. Rev Esp Enferm Dig 2012; 104: 69-71.

[53] Ge ZZ. Efficacy of thalidomide for refractory gastrointestinal bleeding from vascular malformations. Gastroenterology 2011;141:1629-37.

[54] Cushing M. Factor VIII/vonWillebrand Factor Concentrate Therapy for Ventricular-Assist Device associated Acquired vonWillebrand Disease. Transfusion 2012;52:1535-1541

Chapter 4

Allosensitization and the Ventricular Assist Device: Dual Evolution of Technology

Myra Coppage

Additional information is available at the end of the chapter

http://dx.doi.org/10.5772/56426

1. Introduction

Heart failure is a growing worldwide phenomenon, affecting more than 10 million people between the U.S. and Europe [1]. The quality of life for advanced heart failure patients is poor, with repeat hospitalizations and high rates of mortality. With the aging of the general population the number of people experiencing heart failure will rise. Cardiac transplantation has been the goal for some patients, but the growth in number of available donors has not kept pace with the number of potential recipients, and optimal candidates are carefully selected. As a result the search for alternative therapies to support a failing heart, in particular the development of ventricular assist devices (VAD) has been a focus of research for more than 30 years.

Because refractory heart failure frequently involves failure of the dominant left ventricle, early devices were designed to assume the work of the left ventricle. The intent was to improve overall blood flow to the body and organs, reducing some symptoms and secondary end organ failure. Early devices were used primarily as a bridge to transplantation (BTT) to assist patients waiting for a suitable organ. The technology has continued to advance over the last decade and many such devices are in use as stand alone, or destination therapy. The use of VADs has been associated with immune dysregulation and allosensitization, which can be an impediment to transplantation.

This chapter will review the evolution of assist devices in relation to alloimmunity, specifically antibodies to human leukocyte antigens (HLA). The development of antibodies to HLA antigens is caused by exposure via pregnancy, transplantation, and blood transfusion. The level and specificity of alloantibodies is detected by screening against a panel of typed cells or antigen bound to a solid surface, and is reported as panel/percent reactive antibodies (PRA). Different test methods have yield different sensitivity with cell-based (complement dependent cytotoxicity; CDC) being least sensitive and solid phase being most sensitive.

2. Role of alloantibody in acute rejection and chronic allograft vasculopathy

The rapid evolution of effective immunosuppressant drugs has significantly decreased the frequency and severity of acute cellular rejection following cardiac transplantation, but the incidence and effective treatment of antibody mediated rejection (AMR), especially over the long term remains problematic. AMR was first described in 1987 by Herskowitz [2] as arteriolar vasculitis associated with poor outcome. Patients at increased risk are multiparous women and patients with alloantibody against donor antigens detected both pre- and post-transplant. Diagnosis requires clinical graft dysfunction, pathological evidence (endothelial swelling, presence of C4d positive staining on biopsy), and detectable donor specific antibody. Available treatments include plasmapheresis, intravenous steroids, intravenous immunoglobulin, and monoclonal antibodies directed against antibody producing cells (e.g. Rituximab targets CD20).

Acute AMR with high titer antibody damages graft tissue by activation and fixation of complement. The cascade induces coagulation and the terminal event results in the membrane attack complex which injures vascular endothelium. Severe AMR can result in death. Lower titer alloantibody associated with chronic AMR activates endothelial intracellular signaling cascades [3] inducing cell proliferation manifested ultimately as transplant vasculopathy and deterioration of graft function. Ho [4] recently reported results of a large cohort (n=950) of transplants with long term follow-up including biopsies and HLA antibody testing. Development of AMR had significant impact on long term graft survival (16% versus 63% in the AMR negative group at 12 years). In most cases the recipient demonstrated antibody directed against donor HLA antigens. Importantly those who developed antibody more than one year after transplant had the worst outcomes.

Since recipients who demonstrate pretransplant anti-HLA antibodies have higher risk of graft dysfunction, preventing allosensitization is important. However, the use of ventricular assist devices has a history of association with high alloantibody titer. Minimizing the incidence of antibody induction is of prime importance. Table 1 summarizes existing literature of allosensitization among VAD implanted patients. There is a trend toward decreasing allosensitization over time, concurrent with evolution of device from pulsatile to axial flow, evolution of antibody testing from cell-based to solid phase, and an increasing use of leukoreduced blood products.

http://dx.doi.org/10.5772/56426

Author	Study period	Center	Device	n=	PRA>10% (method)	% male	Blood modification
Massad, M et al 1997	1992-1995	Cleveland	HeartMate pulsatile	53	65% (CDC)	87.0%	Few leukoreduced
John R et al, 2003	1992-99	New York	HeartMate pulsatile	105	66% (CDC)	78.1%	Not reported
Drakos, S et al 2007	1993-2002	Utah	HeartMate pulsatile	71	53.7% (CDC)	91.5%	Lower among leukofiltered
McKenna D, et al 2002	1995-2000	Minneapolis	not reported	29	28%	83.0%	Few leukofiltered
Pagani F et al 2000	1996-2000	Michigan	HeartMate pulsatile	38	28% (CDC)	67.6%	Most leukofiltered
George I, et al 2008	1999-2006	New York	HeartMate pulsatile	36	28% (CDC)	83.0%	Most leukofiltered
Arnaoutakis, et al 2011	2004-2009	UNOS	HM XVE pulsatile	673	25.3% (multiple)	84.8%	Not reported
Kumpati, G et al 2004	1991-2000	Cleveland	HM/Novacor pulsatile	231	<5% (CDC)	84.0%	Filtration >1995
Baran, D et al 2005	1989-2002	New Jersey	Novacor pulsatile	26	27% (CDC)	96.2%	Not reported
Kirsch, L et al 2007	1985-2006	Brussels	Novacor pulsatile	27	18.5% (CDC)	65.5%	Not reported
George I, et al 2008	1999-2006	New York	HeartMate II/ DeBakey	24	8% (CDC)	83.0%	Most leukofiltered
Grinda, J et al 2005	199-2004	Paris	DeBakey- axial	14	0% CDC/ELISA	100.0%	All leukoreduced
Drakos, S et al 2009	not reported	Utah	HeartMate II axial	11	9% (CDC/bead array)	63.6%	Most leukofiltered
Coppage, M et al	2009	New York	Mixed multiple	55	8% (CDC/bead array)	85.0%	All leukoreduced

Table 1. Literature on allosensitization among recipients of assist devices.

3. Volume displacement pumps

Early devices were designed to mimic the pulsatile flow of a native heart [5]. These devices include the Thoratec "HeartMate I XVE/1P" and the Abiomed "BVS5000/AB5000." Due to the mechanical nature of these devices reliability was an issue. This first generation of pumps had large surface area that contacted both tissue and blood, and were associated with multiple reports of coagulopathy, immune dysregulation, and allosensitization. In 1997 Massad [6] reported that LVAD (HeartMate) patients were at increased risk for development of antibodies to HLA. While less than 5% of the 53 patients observed had PRA greater than 10% as measured in the CDC assay prior to VAD placement, 66% developed antibody after receiving a VAD.

The overall mean PRA increased significantly from 2.1% to 33.5% during VAD support, although a decrease was observed over time. One source of sensitization to HLA antigens is transfusion, and this group also reported an average of 148 units of blood products on the HeartMate, although the association was limited to transfusion associated with the LVAD and not remote blood product support. During the next few years, other groups also reported that VAD implantation was associated with allosensitization [7-9].

In contrast Stringham [10] reported on a small population (n=6) of recipients who survived VAD implantation without transfusion of blood or platelets. Three of the patients had no history of and did not develop anti-HLA antibody up to transplantation at days 33-50. The other three patients all became highly sensitized with PRA >90% between 30 and 90 days after the VAD surgery. They speculate three potential causes. First, all of the patients did receive fresh frozen plasma (FFP) after separation from the cardiopulmonary bypass, and FFP may contain soluble HLA antigens. Second, two of the three had experienced previous cardiac surgery accompanied by transfusion. They argue that the cardiac dysfunction leading up to VAD placement may have induced a state of immune anergy that was broken when improved cardiac function was restored. This association is not supported by the previously reported Massad[6] study that demonstrated no correlation between remote cardiac surgery with transfusion and later sensitization. Finally, they postulate that immunogenic component(s) of the LVAD cause development of antibody directed against or cross-reactive with HLA antigens. The same group [11] later presented a larger cohort of HeartMate recipient (n=71) analyzing the effect of leuko-reduced blood products, but found no significant effect. Our laboratory [12] reported a series of 55 VAD recipients, most of whom had received a pulsatile device. Our center only uses leuko-reduced, irradiated, and ABO matched blood products and we observed minimal allosensitization.

Drakos [13] undertook a study to determine risk factors contributing to allosensitization. They reviewed records of 75 patients, most of whom received the HeartMate I. The most significant factor identified was a history of prior sensitization to HLA antigens, followed by female gender. Neither of these findings is surprising. Pregnancy is a common sensitizing event, and the presence of HLA allosensitization predisposes to increased antibody production upon re-exposure to antigen. This same group [14] investigated the use of prophylactic intravenous immunoglobulin, commonly used in desensitization strategies, in prevention of HLA sensitization. Patients received either no IVIG or 10g per day of IVIG for 3 days after VAD implantation. The groups were of equal size (25 and 26 respectively), but were not randomized. No statistically significant difference in PRA was observed between the groups, and the overall rate of sensitization (defined as PRA >10%) was over 30% for both.

Several reports addressed the issue of allosensitization stratified by the type of device. The early reports compared the pulsatile pumps with one another. Baran [15] assessed sensitization in a series of 23 patients who received the Novacor (Worldheart, Ottawa) device prior to transplant as opposed to the HeartMate for which previous high PRA had been reported. They note that the HeartMate I was made of textured titanium that develops a neointimal lining that averts the need for systemic anti-coagulation. However, the existence of this lining was suggested to induce immune up-regulation associated with increased PRA. The Novacor had a smooth blood-contacting surface that would not develop a neointimal lining. Of the 23 patients, 13 had less than 5% change in PRA, five had increases of up to 30%, and five experienced a decrease in PRA as tested in the CDC assay. Post-transplant courses were not significantly different between the BTT and non-BTT groups with similar rates of rejection and transplant vasculopathy. Another group [16] undertook a propensity matched study of 231 patients who received either the HeartMate I (n=166) or Novacor (n=55) device. In contrast to Baran [15], this group observed no differential rate of sensitization in a much larger patient population. However, they did report a general rapid, but small increase in PRA in the immediate post-VAD implantation period that decreased over time. In this study, the predictors of sensitization include female sex (pregnancy is a common source of allosensitization) and total number of blood transfusions. The overall level of sensitization of this population was lower than previous reports, with peak PRA <50%, possibly due to their predominant use of leukoreduced blood products.

Gonzalez-Stawinski [17] reviewed early and late rejection as well as HLA sensitization in a series of 119 recipients who were bridged to transplant with 3 different types of VAD, but all were volume displacement. Not surprisingly, higher PRA and positive flow cytometry crossmatch was associated with increased level of rejection on biopsy at 30 days and 2 years post-transplant, but long term outcome was not addressed. However, Joyce [18] surveyed the International Society of Heart and Lung Transplant (ISHLT) registry and divided the cardiac transplant group (n=11,457) into 3 groups including LVAD used, not used, or unknown. Virtually all of the VAD recipients receive pulsatile devices. In this large dataset, the presence of VAD was a significantly higher (p<0.0001) predictor of sensitization as defined by PRA>10%. Importantly, rates of rejection, measured by comparing drug treated events from transplant to 1 year follow up were not different between recipients who bridged with a VAD and those who did not. Likewise there were no significant differences in mortality at 1 or 2 years between the groups.

4. Axial flow pumps

The second generations of assist devices are smaller and contain an impeller that spins to deliver blood through the circulatory system [5]. These pumps are much smaller in size, but the impeller moves at 6000 rpm to 15000 rpm, which may cause hemolysis and platelet activation contributing to general immune activation.

Grinda[19] reported Anti-HLA sensitization for a group of 21 patients who were implanted with the DeBakey axial flow VAD. For this study PRA was measured by both the CDC and solid phase assays. None of their patients developed detectable anti-HLA antibodies during the course of VAD support with mean duration 87 days (range 21-224). This group also uses only leukoreduced blood products. Their findings were supported by a later report from George[20] who compared sensitization observed among patients who received one of two axial flow devices (HeartMate II and DeBakcy n=21) with the pulsatile (HeartMate I n=36) device. Alloantibody was tested in all patients by the CDC method, and sensitization was defined as a PRA of >10%. The actual percent PRA was not reported. They observed a significantly higher rate of sensitization for recipients of the HeartMate I pulsatile device (28%) compared with either axial device (8% $p<0.01$). In both groups the number of allosensitized decreased over time and was lower at the time of heart transplant than as measured after VAD placement. The presence of sensitization did not affect short-term survival in either the axial or pulsatile group.

5. Radial flow devices

The third generation of VADs provides radial or centrifugal flow. In general, they are slightly larger than the axial flow devices, but their design makes them especially suited to long term cardiac support. For that reason these devices are ideal for use as a destination or permanent therapy. Allosensitization would therefore not be an impediment to future therapy. There is one report [21] of successful cardiac transplantation of a small cohort of recipients who had been implanted with HeartWare (Heartware International, USA) or VentriAssist (Ventracor, Ltd, Australia) centrifugal devices. Thirteen patients were transplanted with a one year survival of 91%. While no allosensitization or crossmatch data are presented, one may infer that alloantibody was not a obstruction to transplantation. Conversely, there is a report [22] regarding the Evaheart (Medical USA, Inc) that demonstrates significant platelet activation using centrifugal VAD and two different coatings (carbon versus 2-methoxyethyloylphosphoryl choline) in a bovine model. While platelet activation does not itself lead to allosensitization, platelet activation and microaggreagates were also associated with coagulopathy and ultimately allosensitization in some of the earlier models. As of this writing, no specific reports of anti-HLA antibody associated with the use of radial flow VADs exist.

6. Immune dysregulation associated with VADs

The development of ventricular assist devices provided extended time for patients who were waiting for a compatible heart to become available. The theory and technology has steadily improved over the last 2 decades. Devices are smaller and have a reduced contact with the body's blood and tissue, thus making them less immunogenic. This fact is reflected in the data reviewed here. In the late 1990s and early 2000s, the pulsatile devices were most common, and reports documenting the risk of allosensitization stem from VADs began during this period. The relatively large surface area and composition of materials made for greater contact with tissue and blood, and in addition to reports of allosensitization came reports of general immune dysregulation [23, 24] and coagulopathy [25, 26].

Recipients of the early smooth textured VADs were at increased risk for hemorrhage and later for thromboembolism [27, 28]. Later devices incorporated a textured surface on which developed a neointimal cellular lining. Although the risk of thromboembolic events declined, the cellular lining introduced new complications. These cells were demonstrated to be primarily resting monocytes and activated macrophages[23]. These cells help to maintain an inflammatory state, and were shown to augment production of cytokines (especially of TH2 pathway) and coagulation factors [23]. John [29] studied markers of endothelial and coagulative activation in 21 LVAD recipients (HeartMate II) and noted significant baseline activation of both systems in the immediate postoperative period, with elevated levels remaining to 180 days. Rothenburger [30] also demonstrated that T and NK cell populations decreased and the level remained depressed for over 100 days. At the same time B cell numbers increased as did IL-6 and CRP. Hyper-reactivity of B cells was postulated as VAD recipients demonstrated elevated antiphospholipid antibodies in addition to the risk of anti-HLA antibodies. A more recent study [31] demonstrated the presence of natural antibodies in transplant candidates with VAD. Taken as whole, cardiopulmonary bypass surgery and implantation of a ventricular assist device induces systemic inflammation and humoral amplification[32] including coagulation and complement cascades.

Not surprising given immune dysregulation and the introduction of a foreign body, infection is a nearly universal threat for device-related morbidity. The literature for infectious complications is extensive and will not be reviewed here. The presence of microorganism(s) or fungi, however, contributes to humoral amplification.

7. Immunomodulatory effects of transfused blood products

Our group has observed that soluble immune modulatory factors (sCD40L, IL-8, and RANTES) are present and biologically active in platelet concentrates [33-35] and non-leukoreduced red cells, and to a lesser extent this may be true of FFP as well. We hypothesize that intravenously administered blood components (including FFP), administered as a bolus (as opposed to being produced in a paracrine manner) access the lymphatic system where immune effectors reside, and modulate their responses. This complements previously reported systemic alterations and immune dysregulation involving B cells following VAD implantation [23, 30, 36]. Prior to the general acceptance of universal leukoreduction, a prime indication of this effect on B cell immunity was the production of anti-HLA antibodies. MHC molecules are immunogenic and provide a stimulus for an antibody response. Anti-HLA responses became a focus regarding the hazards of blood transfusion in VAD patients. Immunomodulatory factors present in blood transfusion, especially those that contain white cells or platelets, contribute to a systemic TH2 response, including non-specific activation of B cells and up-regulation of immunoglobulin production [37].

8. Evolution of antibody testing systems

As the technology and understanding of device technology has evolved over the years, so has the science of histocompatibility testing. The practice standard until the last decade was the complement dependent cytotoxicity (CDC) test, often augmented by anti-human globulin

(AHG) to detect low levels of or non-complement fixing antibody. Most of the early reports describe the use of some form of CDC assay, but the addition or exclusion of AHG impacts the sensitivity and specificity of the test. It may allow identification of low level alloantibody, but is also more prone to false positive detection. In the late 1990s, solid-phase assay began to be adapted. The first generation was enzyme-linked immunosorbent assays (ELISA). ELISA assays include HLA antigen bound to a solid, generally plastic surface. These tests are more sensitive than cell based assay, and also include the use of AHG. Newell[38] reported that IgG antibodies detected in the ELISA assay of serum from VAD patients were actually anti-albumin antibodies, a reagent commonly used in ELISA assays. The positive reactions converted to negative when sera were pre-incubated with albumin-coated beads. Similarly, serum from VAD patients tested in our laboratory [12] exhibited reactivity in ELISA assays, but reactivity occurs even in wells that do not contain HLA antigen, indicating false positive reactions.

The up-regulation of humoral immunity described for VAD recipients may include specific (e.g. anti-albumin), non-specific (e.g. natural anti-ABO), and memory (e.g. anti-HLA from pregnancy) antibody responses. Our group has also reported the formation of circulating immune complexes of ABO antigen and their corresponding antibodies in patients who received ABO unmatched platelets [39, 40]. We believe that any or all of these phenomena may interfere with immune assays, especially those that use an anti-immunoglobulin (second-step) reagent such as ELISA, and flow or AHG crossmatch. Recently, however, bead based anti-HLA antibody tests were introduced. In our hands these have proved to be both sensitive and specific, although, like other solid-phase assays they use an anti-human immunoglobulin secondary step. The beads used in these assays are particulate in nature and more rigorous wash steps to remove low avidity antibody may be used to limit weak or non-specific reactions. However, some kits employ recombinant HLA antigen that has an increased propensity for denaturing due to alternate glycosylation and peptide loading. There are multiple reports of "natural" antibody that reacts with HLA antigen [41, 42] and also to denatured HLA antigens [43] that have little or no clinical relevance to allotransplantation. Awareness of the strengths and weaknesses of the various assays that are employed in determining anti-HLA sensitization is vital to accurate interpretation of the data they provide.

A final confounding factor in assessing the role of anti-HLA antibody in ventricular assist devices is how allosensitization is defined. Much of the cardiothoracic literature defines allosensitized as having a PRA > 10%, meaning the candidate has antibody against 10% of the HLA antigens expected among the local organ donor pool. Conversely, this means that the candidate does NOT have antibody to 90% of HLA antigens, and has a 90% likelihood of finding a compatible donor. The histocompatibility community generally does not consider a person highly sensitized unless they demonstrate antibody against more than half of a standard panel. Thus centers who reported rates of sensitization of 30-60% may have simply been using a definition that encompasses patients who should not be so classified. In this light the phenomenon of allosensitization might not exist under a more stringent definition.

In summary, the introduction of a foreign device via major cardiopulmonary bypass surgery is not an immunologically benign event. Patients have systemic complications going into the surgery secondary to cardiac failure. Some of these improve with the introduction of the VAD

http://dx.doi.org/10.5772/56426

and improved blood circulation, but inflammation, infection, and coagulopathy are consistent causes of morbidity and mortality in this population. Continued improvements of the devices to those that are smaller and have continuous flow are less invasive and are more reliable for long term use. Literature around use of the early, large, pulsatile devices pointed to allosensitization to HLA antigens as posing an impediment to using the VAD as a bridge to transplantation. Over the years, our understanding of immune events and the systems used to tests for allosensitization have also evolved. In addition many centers have implemented policies for using leukoreduced blood products. While the development of anti-HLA antibodies is a clear risk for some recipients (e.g. multiparous women, previous sensitized recipients), the phenomenon is not as widespread as once assumed.

Author details

Myra Coppage*

University of Rochester Medical Center, Department of Pathology and Laboratory Medicine, Rochester, NY, USA

References

[1] Roger, V. L, Go, A. S, Lloyd-jones, D. M, Benjamin, E. J, & Berry, J. D. Borden WBet al. : Executive summary: heart disease and stroke statistics--(2012). update: a report from the American Heart Association. Circulation;125:188.

[2] Herskowitz, A, Soule, L. M, Ueda, K, Tamura, F, & Baumgartner, W. A. Borkon AMet al. : Arteriolar vasculitis on endomyocardial biopsy: a histologic predictor of poor outcome in cyclosporine-treated heart transplant recipients. J Heart Transplant (1987).

[3] Zhang, X. Reed EF: Effect of Antibodies on Endothelium. American Journal of Transplantation (2009).

[4] Ho, E. K, Vlad, G, Vasilescu, E. R, De La Torre, L, & Colovai, A. I. Burke Eet al. : Pre- and posttransplantation allosensitization in heart allograft recipients: Major impact of de novo alloantibody production on allograft survival. Human Immunology (2011).

[5] Timms, D. A review of clinical ventricular assist devices. Medical Engineering & Physics;33:1041.

[6] Massad, M. G, Cook, D. J, Schmitt, S. K, Smedira, N. G, & Mccarthy, J. F. Vargo RLet al. : Factors influencing HLA sensitization in implantable LVAD recipients. Ann Thorac Surg (1997).

[7] Pagani, F. D, Dyke, D. B, Wright, S, & Cody, R. Aaronson KD: Development of anti-major histocompatibility complex class I or II antibodies following left ventricular assist device implantation: effects on subsequent allograft rejection and survival. J Heart Lung Transplant (2001).

[8] Mckenna, D. H. Jr., Eastlund T, Segall M, Noreen HJ, Park S: HLA alloimmunization in patients requiring ventricular assist device support. J Heart Lung Transplant (2002).

[9] John, R, Lietz, K, Schuster, M, Naka, Y, & Rao, V. Mancini DMet al. : Immunologic sensitization in recipients of left ventricular assist devices. J Thorac Cardiovasc Surg (2003).

[10]]Stringham, J. C, Bull, D. A, Fuller, T. C, Kfoury, A. G, & Taylor, D. O. Renlund DGet al. : Avoidance of cellular blood product transfusions in LVAD recipients does not prevent HLA allosensitization. J Heart Lung Transplant (1999).

[11]]Drakos, S. G, Stringham, J. C, Long, J. W, Gilbert, E. M, & Fuller, T. C. Campbell BKet al. : Prevalence and risks of allosensitization in HeartMate left ventricular assist device recipients: the impact of leukofiltered cellular blood product transfusions. J Thorac Cardiovasc Surg (2007).

[12] Coppage, M, Baker, M, Fialkow, L, Meehan, D, & Gettings, K. Chen Let al. : Lack of significant de novo HLA allosensitization in ventricular assist device recipients transfused with leukoreduced, ABO identical blood products. Hum Immunol (2009).

[13] Drakos, S. G, Kfoury, A. G, Kotter, J. R, Reid, B. B, & Clayson, S. E. Selzman CHet al. : Prior human leukocyte antigen-allosensitization and left ventricular assist device type affect degree of post-implantation human leukocyte antigen-allosensitization. J Heart Lung Transplant (2009).

[14] Drakos, S. G, Kfoury, A. G, Long, J. W, Stringham, J. C, & Fuller, T. C. Nelson KEet al. : Low-dose prophylactic intravenous immunoglobulin does not prevent HLA sensitization in left ventricular assist device recipients. Ann Thorac Surg (2006).

[15] Baran, D. A, Gass, A. L, Galin, I. D, Zucker, M. J, & Arroyo, L. H. Goldstein DJet al. : Lack of Sensitization and Equivalent Post-transplant Outcomes With the Novacor Left Ventricular Assist Device. The Journal of Heart and Lung Transplantation (2005).

[16] Kumpati, G. S, Cook, D. J, Blackstone, E. H, Rajeswaran, J, & Abdo, A. S. Young JBet al. : HLA sensitization in ventricular assist device recipients: does type of device make a difference? J Thorac Cardiovasc Surg (2004).

[17] Gonzalez-stawinski, G. V, Atik, F. A, Mccarthy, P. M, Roselli, E. E, & Hoercher, K. Navia JLet al. : Early and late rejection and HLA sensitization at the time of heart transplantation in patients bridged with left ventricular assist devices. Transplant Proc (2005).

[18] Joyce, D. L, Southard, R. E, Torre-amione, G, Noon, G. P, & Land, G. A. Loebe M: Impact of Left Venticular Assist Device (LVAD)-mediated Humoral Sensitization on Post-transplant Outcomes. The Journal of Heart and Lung Transplantation (2005).

[19] Grinda, J. M, Bricourt, M. O, Amrein, C, Salvi, S, & Guillemain, R. Francois Aet al. : Human leukocyte antigen sensitization in ventricular assist device recipients: a lesser risk with the DeBakey axial pump. Ann Thorac Surg (2005).

[20] George, I, Colley, P, Russo, M. J, Martens, T. P, & Burke, E. Oz MCet al. : Association of device surface and biomaterials with immunologic sensitization after mechanical support. The Journal of Thoracic and Cardiovascular Surgery (2008).

[21] Kutty, R. S, Parameshwar, J, Lewis, C, Catarino, P. A, & Sudarshan, C. D. Jenkins DPet al. : Use of centrifugal left ventricular assist device as a bridge to candidacy in severe heart failure with secondary pulmonary hypertension. European Journal of Cardio-Thoracic Surgery (2013).

[22] Snyder, T. A, Tsukui, H, Kihara, S, Akimoto, T, & Litwak, K. N. Kameneva MVet al. : Preclinical biocompatibility assessment of the EVAHEART ventricular assist device: coating comparison and platelet activation. J Biomed Mater Res A (2007).

[23] Itescu, S. John R: Interactions between the recipient immune system and the left ventricular assist device surface: immunological and clinical implications. Ann Thorac Surg (2003). S58.

[24] Thompson, L. O, & Loebe, M. Noon GP: What price support? Ventricular assist device induced systemic response. ASAIO J (2003).

[25] Himmelreich, G, Ullmann, H, Riess, H, Rosch, R, & Loebe, M. Schiessler Aet al. : Pathophysiologic role of contact activation in bleeding followed by thromboembolic complications after implantation of a ventricular assist device. ASAIO J (1995). M790.

[26] Spanier, T, Oz, M, Levin, H, Weinberg, A, & Stamatis, K. Stern Det al. : Activation of coagulation and fibrinolytic pathways in patients with left ventricular assist devices. J Thorac Cardiovasc Surg (1996).

[27] Kasirajan, V, Mccarthy, P. M, Hoercher, K. J, Starling, R. C, & Young, J. B. Banbury MKet al. : Clinical experience with long-term use of implantable left ventricular assist devices: indications, implantation, and outcomes. Semin Thorac Cardiovasc Surg (2000).

[28] Portner, P. M, Jansen, P. G, Oyer, P. E, & Wheeldon, D. R. Ramasamy N: Improved outcomes with an implantable left ventricular assist system: a multicenter study. Ann Thorac Surg (2001).

[29] John, R, Panch, S, Hrabe, J, Wei, P, & Solovey, A. Joyce Let al. : Activation of Endothelial and Coagulation Systems in Left Ventricular Assist Device Recipients. The Annals of Thoracic Surgery (2009).

[30] Rothenburger, M, Wilhelm, M, Hammel, D, Schmid, C, & Plenz, G. Tjan TDet al. : Immune response in the early postoperative period after implantation of a left-ventricular assist device system. Transplant Proc (2001).

[31] Nikaein, A, Awar, N, Hunt, J, Rosenthal, E. J, & Eichhorn, E. Hall Set al. : Clinically irrelevant circulating human leukocyte antigen antibodies in the presence of ventricular assist devices. J Heart Lung Transplant;31:443.

[32] Kirklin, J. K, Westaby, S, Blackstone, E. H, Kirklin, J. W, & Chenoweth, D. E. Pacifico AD: Complement and the damaging effects of cardiopulmonary bypass. J Thorac Cardiovasc Surg (1983).

[33] Blumberg, N, Gettings, K. F, Turner, C, & Heal, J. M. Phipps RP: An association of soluble CD40 ligand (CD154) with adverse reactions to platelet transfusions. Transfusion (2006).

[34] Kaufman, J, Spinelli, S. L, Schultz, E, & Blumberg, N. Phipps RP: Release of biologically active CD154 during collection and storage of platelet concentrates prepared for transfusion. J Thromb Haemost (2007).

[35] Khan, S. Y, Kelher, M. R, Heal, J. M, Blumberg, N, & Boshkov, L. K. Phipps Ret al. : Soluble CD40 ligand accumulates in stored blood components, primes neutrophils through CD40, and is a potential cofactor in the development of transfusion-related acute lung injury. Blood (2006).

[36] Hampton, C. R. Verrier ED: Systemic consequences of ventricular assist devices: alterations of coagulation, immune function, inflammation, and the neuroendocrine system. Artif Organs (2002).

[37] Rothenburger, M, Wilhelm, M, Hammel, D, Schmid, C, & Plenz, G. Tjan TDTet al. : Immune response in the early postoperative period after implantation of a left-ventricular assist device system. Transplantation Proceedings (2001).

[38] Newell, H, Smith, J. D, Rogers, P, Birks, E, & Danskine, A. J. Fawson REet al. : Sensitization following LVAD implantation using leucodepleted blood is not due to HLA antibodies. Am J Transplant (2006).

[39] Heal, J. M, & Masel, D. Blumberg N: Interaction of platelet fc and complement receptors with circulating immune complexes involving the AB0 system. Vox Sang (1996).

[40] Heal, J. M, Masel, D, & Rowe, J. M. Blumberg N: Circulating immune complexes involving the ABO system after platelet transfusion. Br J Haematol (1993).

[41] Morales-buenrostro, L. E, Terasaki, P. I, Marino-vazquez, L. A, Lee, J. H, & Awar, N. Alberu J: "Natural" human leukocyte antigen antibodies found in nonalloimmunized healthy males. Transplantation (2008).

[42] El-Awar, N, Terasaki, P. I, Cai, J, Deng, C. T, & Ozawa, M. Nguyen Aet al. : Epitopes of HLA-A, B, C, DR, DQ, DP and MICA antigens. Clin Transpl (2009).

[43] Poli, F, Benazzi, E, Innocente, A, Nocco, A, & Cagni, N. Gianatti Aet al. : Heart transplantation with donor-specific antibodies directed toward denatured HLA-A*02:01: a case report. Hum Immunol (2011).

Chapter 5

Preliminary Trial of Lower Leg Thermal Therapy for Patients with Terminal Heart Failure Fitted with Left Ventricular Assist Device

Kazuo Komamura, Toshiaki Shishido and Takeshi Nakatani

Additional information is available at the end of the chapter

http://dx.doi.org/10.5772/55819

1. Introduction

In 1989 Tei et al. developed Waon therapy for heart failure that uses a dry sauna (Tei et al., 1994; Tei et al., 1995; Tei 2007). Waon therapy means a thermal therapy using specially designed sauna bath for heart failure. In the therapy, patients were placed in a sitting-position in a 60 ∘C far infrared-ray dry sauna system for 15 min, and then after leaving the sauna, they underwent bed rest with a blanket to keep them warm for an additional 30 min. And fluids corresponding to perspiration are supplied to protect against dehydration at the end of therapy. In this specially designed sauna system, the body core temperature has increased by 1.0–1.2°C, various beneficial effects for symptoms of heart failure were found (Tei, 2007).

Tei et al. have reported that Waon therapy significantly improved clinical symptoms, increased ejection fraction, and decreased cardiac size on echocardiography and chest radiography in congestive heart failure (CHF) patients (Tei & Tanaka, 1996). Recently, Miyata M et al. confirmed the beneficial effects and safety of Waon therapy applied for 2 weeks in CHF patients in a prospective multicenter case—control study (Miyata et al., 2008). Kihara et al. previously demonstrated that Waon therapy improved not only cardiac function, but also endothelial function in patients with CHF. They have also reported that 2 weeks of Waon therapy significantly reduced brain natriuretic peptide blood levels and improved flow-mediated vasodilation in CHF patients (Kihara et al., 2002). Furthermore, they have reported that Waon therapy for 2 weeks decreased ventricular premature contractions and increased heart rate variability in CHF patients (Kihara et al., 2004), suggesting that Waon therapy decreased sympathetic nervous activity and improved ventricular arrhythmias.

A large number of end-stage CHF patients in Japan have been implanted with a left ventricular assist device (LVAD) because of prolonged waiting period for heart transplants (Osada et al., 2005). Although we wished to apply sauna thermal therapy to patients with LVAD, we do not have an appropriate sauna facility. Thus, we attempted to apply lower leg thermal therapy to the patients with LVAD awaiting a heart transplant. We describe here a case series of lower leg thermal therapy for the first time to elucidate the safety and effectiveness of this preliminary trial for the patients fitted with left ventricular assist device for end-stage heart failure.

2. Methods

2.1. Patients and study design

The study subjects included consecutive 6 end-stage CHF patients who were listed on waiting list for heart transplant in National Cerebral and Cardiovascular Center, Suita, Japan. All patients had dilated cardiomyopathy refractory to maximal medical therapy including angiotensin-converting enzyme inhibitors or angiotensin receptor blockers, beta-blockers, diuretics, and digitalis. Regardless of intensive care with intravenous inotropic agents, heart failure rapidly progressed to cardiogenic shock in the patients. And they were fitted with extracorporeal LVAD (VCT-50, Toyobo Ltd., Osaka, Japan) to stabilize the hemodynamics. None of the patients was implanted with a defibrillator device.

Patients' general condition stabilized thereafter and the status of heart failure at the time of study was New York Heart Association (NYHA) class IIm with hemodynamic support. Although this status remained stable for at least 6 months, patients' cardiac function did not sufficiently recover to discontinue LVAD support. The patient provided written informed consent to enter into a clinical trial of lower leg thermal therapy for patients with LVAD awaiting a heart transplant. The Ethics Committee at the National Cerebral and Cardiovascular Center approved the protocol, and the study was conducted in accordance with the Declaration of Helsinki. Lower leg thermal therapy was conducted with a steam bath at 42 ∘C. Typical example of lower leg thermal therapy was illustrated in Fig.1.

After 15 min of therapy at 42 ∘C, the patient remained seated in the steam bath with the lower legs and feet wrapped with a blanket for 30 min. The study consisted of clinical examinations before and after daily thermal therapy for 2 weeks (Fig. 2).

Study protocol for 2 weeks treatment was illustrated in Fig. 3. The procedure of lower leg thermal therapy was accompanied by electrocardiographic monitoring. The patient remained on the same medications with same dose throughout the study period.

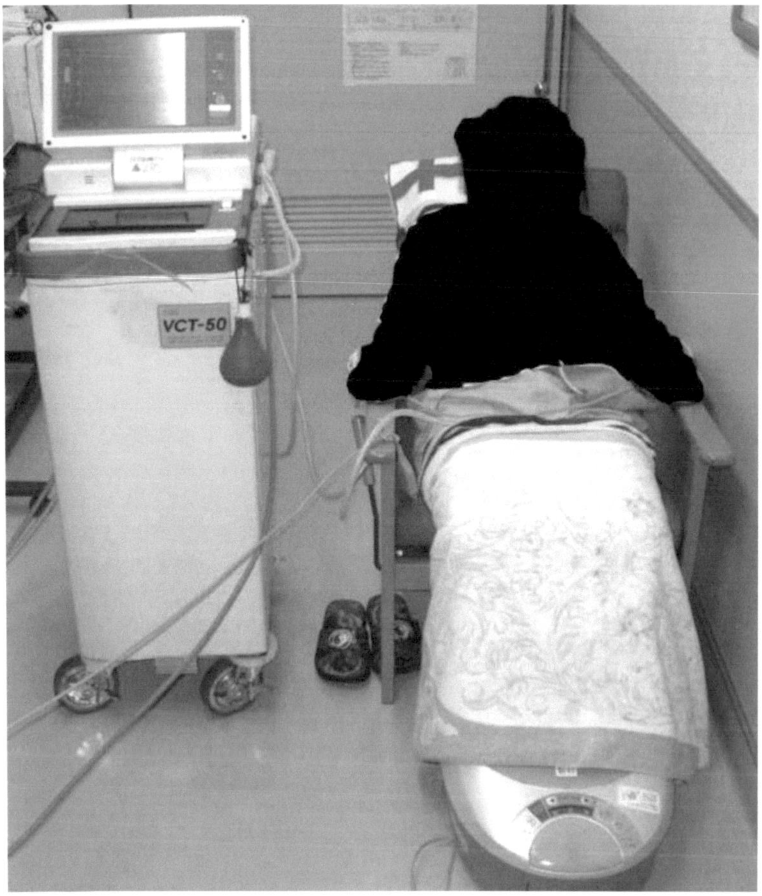

Figure 1. Typical settings for lower leg thermal therapy for a patient with left ventricular assist device.

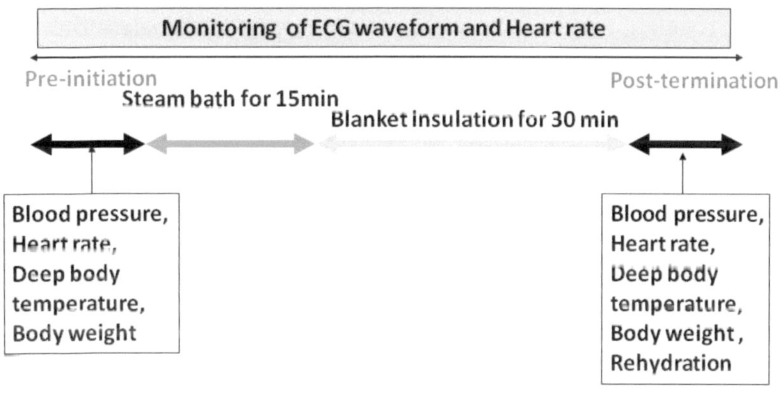

Figure 2. Illustrative presentation of the lower leg thermal therapy.

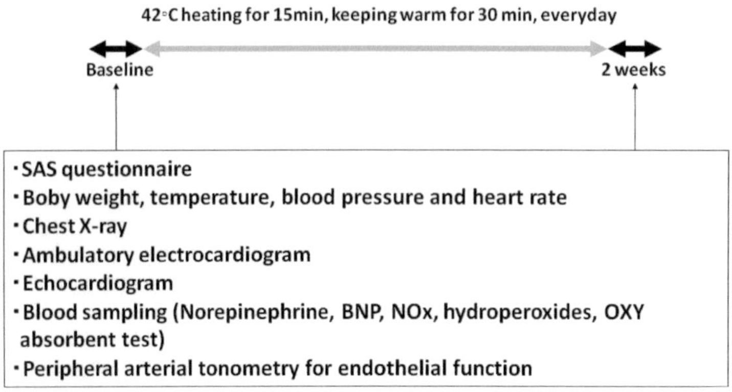

Figure 3. Illustrative presentation of the study design of lower leg thermal therapy.

2.2. Measurements

Systolic and diastolic blood pressure (BP), heart rate, body weight, surface and deep body temperature (axillary and sublingual) were measured everyday throughout the study. Chest X-ray, ambulatory electrocardiogram, echocardiogram and peripheral arterial tonometry were recorded and blood sampling was taken before and 2 weeks after the treatment. Blood sampling was used for measurement of plasma BNP, plasma nitrates and nitrites, plasma hydroperoxides, and HClO expense test.

Medical interview was done every morning to evaluate clinical status of CHF by NYHA functional class, and to estimate patients' activity of daily life using Specific Activity Scale (SAS). We used the Specific Activity Scale as a measure of quality of life (QOL) in which self-perceived exercise tolerance is expressed by an energy cost spent in the maximal physical activity that the patient can perform (Sasayama et al., 1992). The Specific Activity Scale allows expression of the extent of submaximal physical activity. Sasayama et al. actually measured the metabolic costs of various types of physical activity by hooking subjects up to a mask to measure oxygen consumption and the volume of carbon dioxide exhaled. Then they prepared questionnaires about specific physical activities that a patient would perform either customarily or sporadically in daily life and each patient was asked to specify whether he/she could perform each type of activity without symptomatic limitation. Summarizing the questionnaire data, a given number of metabolic costs (Specific Activity Scale) were derived for each patient with regard to the self-perceived exercise tolerance. As a clear linear correlation was observed between Specific Activity Scale and peak oxygen consumption, the Specific Activity Scale was considered to reliably predict exercise capacity (Sasayama et al., 1992)

Before and 2 weeks after the treatment, the cardiothoracic ratio (CTR) was measured by chest radiography and daily count of ventricular premature beats was evaluated with ambulatory electrocardiogram. Before and 2 weeks after the treatment, two-dimensional echocardiography were performed to determine left ventricular systolic (LVDs) and diastolic dimension (LVDd), left atrial dimension (LAD), LV fractional shortening and degree of mitral regurgitation.

Venous blood samples were drawn through an indwelling catheter in the forearm of each patient after they had lain quietly and undisturbed for at least 30 min. Plasma was immediately separated and stored at –70°C before the norepinephrine (NE) concentrations were determined by high performance liquid chromatography electrochemical detection. Plasma brain natriuretic peptide (BNP) was determined by the chemiluminescent enzyme immunoassay. For nitric oxide (NO) measurement, the blood specimen was placed immediately in an ice bath and centrifuged within 30 seconds for 5 minutes at 2000*g*. The serum fraction was diluted 1:1 with nitrite- and nitrate-free distilled water, and 400 mL of the diluted sample was centrifuged at 2000*g* in an ultra-free MC microcentrifuge device (Millipore) to remove substances larger than 10 kD. The filtrate was passed through a copper-plated cadmium column to reduce nitrate to nitrite and then reacted with Griess reagents consisting of 0.1% naphthylethylenediamine dihydrochloride in distilled water and 1% sulfanilamide in 5% H_3PO_4, after which absorbance was measured at 540 nm to provide the total amount of plasma NO end products (nitrate plus nitrite). The efficiency of the cadmium column in the conversion of nitrate to nitrite was confirmed to be 100% by measuring both nitrate and nitrite standards before and after sample measurement (Node et al., 1997). Plasma hydroperoxides, which was determined by Diacron reactive oxygen metabolites test, comprise a marker of oxidative stress (Cesarone et al., 1999) and OXY absorbent test indicates buffering potential against oxidant action of hypochlorous acid (HClO), which is quantified by HClO expense, and comprise a marker of anti-oxidative potency (Trotti et al., 2001).

Endothelial function was quantified by the reactive hyperemic (RH) change in digital blood flow after arm occlusion using a peripheral fingertip arterial tonometry (PAT) device (Endo-PAT 2000 system; Itamar-Medical, Caesarea, Israel) (Bonetti et al., 2004; Hamburg & Benjamin, 2009). After 5 min of baseline recording, a BP cuff was inflated to supra-systolic pressure in the test arm. After 5 min of occlusion, the cuff was rapidly deflated, with PAT tracings recorded. The reactive hyperemic PAT (RH-PAT) response was determined as the ratio of PAT amplitude in the test arm to control arm, averaged in 30-s intervals after cuff deflation, divided by the average PAT ratio measured for the 140-s interval before cuff inflation. RH-PAT ratio was assessed between 60 s and 120 s after occlusion and was log-transformed of the post-deflation to baseline pulse amplitude in the hyperemic finger normalized to the contralateral finger.

2.3. Statistical analysis

All data are expressed as the mean value±S.D. Differences between the baseline and 2 weeks after treatment were estimated by paired t test or Mann–Whitney U test, as appropriate for continuous variables, and by Fisher's exact test or chi square test, as appropriate for categorical variables. Value of BNP was log-transformed to remove skewness of data distribution. A *p*-value of <0.05 was considered statistically significant.

3. Results

3.1. Clinical findings and physical examinations

Table 1 summarized the results of clinical findings and physical examinations. During the study, none of the patients treated with lower leg thermal therapy had worsened clinical symptoms. The changes in the clinical findings and variables after 2 weeks are summarized in Table. Although NYHA functional class remained similar at class IIm, activity of daily life estimated by SAS system significantly increased from 2.55 Mets to 3.10 Mets ($p = 0.044$).

Systolic and diastolic blood pressure did not differ between the baseline and 2 weeks after the therapy. Heart rate might tend to decrease a little bit from 74 bpm to 72 bpm ($p = 0.088$). Numbers of ventricular premature beats were dispersed among the patients at the baseline as well as 2 weeks after treatment. Thus, the average number of ventricular premature beats was not different between the baseline and 2 weeks after the therapy.

There was no significant change in body weight. Body surface temperature (axillary temperature) in the morning round was not different between the baseline and 2 weeks after the therapy. However, the deep body temperature (sublingual temperature) significantly increased from 36.0 degree Celsius to 36.9 degree Celsius ($p = 0.004$), just after the steam bath for lower legs. The average difference between the baseline and immediately after the therapy was 0.85 degree Celsius.

	Before	**After**	**p value**
Sample size	6	6	
Age (years)	34.8±8.0		
Activity of Daily Life (Mets)	2.55±0.81	3.10±0.99	0.044
Systolic BP (mmHg)	91.2±10.0	92.3±14.4	0.682
Diastolic BP (mmHg)	54.8±9.0	56.8±9.2	0.310
Heart Rate (bpm)	74.0±8.3	71.9±8.3	0.088
Ventricular Premature Beats (per day)	92.8±48.1	55.3±15.9	0.100
Body Weight (kg)	53.2±8.9	53.0±9.2	0.383
Morning Body Temperature (C)	35.8±0.33	36.0±0.41	0.476
Deep Body Temperature (C)	36.0±0.26	36.9±0.36	0.004
Cardiothoracic Ratio (%)	56.6±13.2	55.3±13.7	0.065
NE (pg/mL)	971.2±403.6	848.6±313.5	0.077
log BNP (pg/mL)	2.128±0.516	2.080±0.505	0.030
Nitrogen oxide (μmol/L)	30.1±12.1	46.5±17.7	0.019
Hydroperoxides (carr U)	513.0±75.0	439.3±78.4	0.0001
OXY absorbent test (μmol HCl/mL)	400.7±38.2	456.7±51.9	0.078
LAD (mm)	43.3±9.4	41.9±9.5	0.063
LVDd (mm)	54.4±10.8	53.1±11.9	0.130
LVDs (mm)	43.2±13.6	40.3±13.8	0.025
LV Fractional Shortening (%)	21.9±8.7	25.3±8.9	0.028
Mitral Regurgitation (grade)	2.2±1.0	1.3±0.8	0.061
RH-PAT ratio	1.36±0.22	2.09±0.28	0.006

BNP brain natriuretic peptide, BP blood pressure, LAD left atrial dimension, LV left ventricular, LVDd left ventricular diastolic diameter, LVDs left ventricular systolic diameter, NE norepinephrine, OXY oxidant, RH-PAT reactive hyperemic peripheral arterial tonometry

Table 1. Summary of changes in parameters before and after the thermal therapy

3.2. Chest radiography and echocardiography

Table 1. described the results of chest radiography and echocardiography. Chest radiography showed a slight decrease of the mean CTR from 57% to 55% after 2 weeks of treatment compared to the baseline ($p = 0.065$).

Echocardiography demonstrated a slight decrease in the mean LAD from 43 mm to 42 mm ($p = 0.063$). While, LVDd showed no changes after treatment (54 mm to 53mm, $p = 0.130$), LVDs significantly decreased after treatment from 43 mm to 40 mm ($p = 0.025$). Therefore, LV fractional shortening also significantly increased after treatment from 22% to 25% ($p = 0.028$).

Doppler echocardiography demonstrated that the extent of mitral regurgitation tended to decrease after treatment (mean MR grade: 2.2 to 1.3, $p = 0.061$). Taken together, the left ventricular function was improved and the heart size tended to decrease after 2 weeks of the therapy.

3.3. plasma levels of norepinephrine, BNP, nitrogen oxide and hydroperoxides, and result of OXY adsorbent test

Table 1. showed the changes in plasma concentration of norepinephrine, BNP, nitrogen oxide (nitrate plus nitrite), hydroperoxides and hypochlorous acid. Plasma mean concentration of norepinephrine slightly decreased after 2 weeks of the therapy (971 pg/mL to 849 pg/mL, $p = 0.077$). The plasma mean concentration of BNP significantly decreased after 2 weeks of the therapy, (log BNP: 2.128 to 2.080 pg/mL, $p = 0.030$).

Plasma mean concentration of nitrogen oxide (nitrate plus nitrite), stable metabolites of nitric oxide, significantly increased after 2 weeks of the therapy (30.1 μmol/L to 46.5 μmol/L, $p = 0.019$). Plasma mean concentration of hydroperoxides, a biomarker reflects oxidative stress, significantly decreased after 2 weeks of the therapy (513 carr U to 439 carr U, $p = 0.0001$). OXY absorbent test, a marker of anti-oxidative potency, showed non-significant increase after 2 weeks of the therapy (401 μmol HClO/mL to 457 μmol HClO/mL, $p = 0.078$)

3.4. Endothelial function

The mean RH-PAT ratio determined with Endo-PAT 2000 system was augmented 2 weeks after the therapy compared to the baseline (1.36 to 2.09, $p = 0.006$).

4. Discussion

This is the first report of case series of lower leg thermal therapy being applied to patients implanted with LVAD and awaiting heart transplantation. Waon therapy or whole body sauna therapy for CHF is now widely recognized to improve clinical symptoms, cardiac function, quality of life, and ventricular arrhythmia, and decreased levels of abnormally activated neurohumoral factors (Tei et al., 1995; Tei & Tanaka, 1996; Tei 2007; Kihara et al., 2002; Kihara et al., 2004).

Waon therapy is impractical for patients with CHF in usual general hospitals that lack sauna facilities, whereas lower leg thermal therapy using a steam bath can be applied routinely in a patient's room in common general hospitals. Increases in deep body temperature of 1.0-1.2 ∘C during Waon therapy dilate systemic arteries and veins, and reduce systemic preload and afterload, resulting in increased cardiac output (Tei et al., 1995; Tei & Tanaka, 1996; Tei 2007; Kihara et al., 2002; Kihara et al., 2004). The sublingual temperature of the patients after our lower leg thermal therapy increased by only 0.85 ∘C. Nevertheless, the clinical benefits seemed to be similar to those of Waon or whole body sauna therapy.

Ikeda et al. found that repeated Waon therapy increases endothelial nitric oxide synthase expression and nitric oxide production, and improves cardiac function in animal models of heart failure (Ikeda et al., 2001; Ikeda et al., 2005). Serum nitrate plus nitrite levels doubled in our patient compared with the baseline values, as did the index of endothelial function determined by RH-PAT. Thus, lower leg thermal therapy might upregulate nitric oxide production in the endothelium.

Recently, Kuwahata et al. demonstrated that Waon therapy suppressed the elevated autonomic nervous activity levels in chronic heart failure (Kuwahata et al., 2011). Fujita et al. reported that Waon therapy reduced oxidative stresses in chronic heart failure (Fujita et al., 2011). Those findings dovetail with the results of the present study. Lower leg thermal therapy may have a stress-reducing effect.

Bating in hot water might supress oxidative stress and enhance endothelial function via upregulation of expression of heat shock protein (Okada M et al., 2004). Immersion not in hot water but in warm water (33-34 ∘C) still ameriorated cardiac dysfunction of chronic heart failure (Cider A et al., 2006). Thus, heating may have a beneficial effects on symptoms of heart failure.

Patients implanted with an LVAD for a long period often develop serious hemorrhage in the cerebrum or elsewhere, and drive-line infections. We were concerned that lower leg thermal therapy would aggravate hemorrhage or infection of patients through its vasodilatory effects. On the contrary, we found that oozing of blood at the insertion site of the LVAD drive-line tended to resolve during the therapy in several patients (data not shown). Furthermore a previous study reported that topical thermal therapy was not expected to be accompanied by marked alterations in heart rate, mean arterial pressure, or cardiac output and therefore would not likely activate the renin-angiotensin aldosterone system (Weber AA et al., 2007). In our present study, we did not find significant changes in hemodynamics of the patients.

Impacts of lower leg exercise on muscles and vessels of lower extrimities ameriolates dyspnea in CHF or chronic obstructive pulmonary disease (Beniaminovitz A et al., 2002; Sillen MJ et al., 2009). And lower leg exercise increased endothelial function even in upper armes and affected clinical symptoms of CHF especially in those who cannot do conventional excercise programme (Deftereos S et al., 2010). Excercise in CHF enhances not only endothelial functions in systemic vasculature but also has anti-inflammatory effects on the endothelium (Duscha BD et al., 2008).

http://dx.doi.org/10.5772/55819

Aside from exercise, heat is a natural vasodilator. Thus, judicious use of heat in the form of thermal baths, saunas, and/or heating pads is slowly gaining recognition as a potential supplement to pharmaceuticals to improve endothelial function and cardiorenal hemodynamics in selected patients with CHF. Yoon et al. reported that warm footbath increased coronary blood flow velocity in the left anterior descending coronary artery by 17% in patients with coronary artery disease (CAD) (Yoon SJ et al., 2011). In our experiment, coronary blood flow velocity in the left anterior descending coronary artery before and after the lower leg thermal therapy was determined in a patient with CHF and the velocity increased by 10% after the therapy (data not shown).

We did not conduct lower leg thermal therapy for CAD patients yet. Previous studies showed the thermal therapy for CAD might cause myocardial ischemia (Giannetti N et al., 1999), or myocardial infarction and sudden cardiac death (Hannuksela ML et al., 2001). Thus, CHF due to non-ischemic diseases like dilated cardiomyopathy in our case might be a good indication for lower leg thermal therapy.

Waon therapy attenuates psychological stress (Kihara et al., 2004). Because of a donor shortage in Japan, patients must remain attached to an LVAD and stay for over 2 years in hospital while waiting for a heart transplant (Takatani et al., 2005). The tendency of decrease in plasma norepinephrine in the present study indicated that lower leg thermal therapy also might attenuate psychological, as well as physical stress.

Compared to pharmacological vasodilator therapy and other non-pharmacological therapy, such as cardiac resynchronization therapy (CRT) or cardiac rehabilitation, there are several advantages of lower leg thermal therapy for CHF. First, it is quite safe and has no adverse effects. Second, it might be less expensive and more cost-effective compared to Waon therapy or CRT. Third, unlike cardiac rehabilitation, patients who have severe congestive heart failure, uncontrolled ventricular arrhythmias, or orthopedic limitations are not exempt from undergoing lower leg thermal therapy. Fourth, this treatment may promote mental and physical relaxation. Above all, the most distinctive feature of lower leg thermal therapy is a potential to be useful in conjunction with other therapeutic modalities of pharmacological and non-pharmacological measures. Lower leg thermal therapy may thus be a valuable adjunct to pharmacological or non-pharmacological intervention in the management of CHF. We have a high expectation for the future of lower leg thermal therapy. All that we need is a randomized clinical trial.

5. Study limitation

Although the present study is just preliminary one, sample size is very small, and is not randomized. Recruitment of study subjects is still continuing. In the present protocol, study subjects were implanted with LVAD for end-stage heart failure, who were not common in usual hospitals. Furthermore, the endpoints are surrogate ones. Thus, we have to be very careful to interpret the study results.

6. Conclusion

Although in a very small cohort, we confirmed that lower leg thermal therapy was quite safe, and improved clinical symptoms and cardiac function in patients with extracorporeal LVAD awaiting heart transplantation. Lower leg thermal therapy may be a valuable adjunct to pharmacological or non-pharmacological intervention in the management of chronic heart failure. The procedure of lower leg thermal therapy might benefit other kinds of patients, including those with end-stage heart failure.

Author details

Kazuo Komamura[1], Toshiaki Shishido[2] and Takeshi Nakatani[2]

1 Cardiovascular Division, Hyogo College of Medicine, Nishinomiya, Japan

2 Division of Heart Failure and Division of Transplantation, National Cerebral and Cardiovascular Center, Suita, Japan

References

[1] Beniaminovitz A, Lang CC, LaManca J, Mancini DM. (2002) Selective low-level leg muscle training alleviates dyspnea in patients with heart failure. *J Am Coll Cardiol* 40:1602-8

[2] Bonetti PO, Pumper GM, Higano ST, Holmes Jr DR, Kuvin JT, Lerman A. (2004) Noninvasive identification of patients with early coronary atherosclerosis by assessment of digital reactive hyperemia. J Am Coll Cardiol 44:2137-41.

[3] Cesarone MR, Belcaro G, Carratelli M, Cornelli U, De Sanctis MT, Incandela L, Barsotti A, Terranova R, Nicolaides A. (1999) A simple test to monitor oxidative stress. *Int Angiol* 18:127-30.

[4] Cider A, Sveälv BG, Täng MS, Schaufelberger M, Andersson B. (2006) Immersion in warm water induces improvement in cardiac function in patients with chronic heart failure. *Eur J Heart Fail* 8:308-13.

[5] Deftereos S, Giannopoulos G, Raisakis K, Kossyvakis C, Kaoukis A, Driva M, Pappas L, Panagopoulou V, Ntzouvara O, Karavidas A, Pyrgakis V, Rentoukas I, Aggeli C, Stefanadis C. (2010) Comparison of muscle functional electrical stimulation to conventional bicycle exercise on endothelium and functional status indices in patients with heart failure. *Am J Cardiol* 106:1621-5.

[6] Duscha BD, Schulze PC, Robbins JL, Forman DE. (2008) Implications of chronic heart failure on peripheral vasculature and skeletal muscle before and after exercise training. *Heart Fail Rev* 13:21-37.

[7] Fujita S, Ikeda Y, Miyata M, Shinsato T, Kubozono T, Kuwahata S, Hamada N, Miyauchi T, Yamaguchi T, Torii H, Hamasaki S, Tei C. (2011) Effect of Waon therapy on oxidative stress in chronic heart failure. *Circ J.* 75(2):348-56.

[8] Giannetti N, Juneau M, Arsenault A, Behr MA, Grégoire J, Tessier M, Larivée L. (1999) Sauna-induced myocardial ischemia in patients with coronary artery disease. *Am J Med* 107:228-33.

[9] Hamburg NM, Benjamin EJ. (2009) Assessment of endothelial function using digital pulse amplitude tonometry. Trends Cardiovasc Med 2009;19:6-11.

[10] Hannuksela ML, Ellahham S. (2001) Benefits and risks of sauna bathing. *Am J Med* 110:118-26.

[11] Ikeda Y, Biro S, Kamogawa Y, Yoshifuku S, Eto H, Orihara K, Kihara T, Tei C. (2001) Repeated thermal therapy upregulates arterial endothelial nitric oxide synthase expression in Syrian golden hamsters. *Jpn Circ J* 65:434-8.

[12] Ikeda Y, Biro S, Kamogawa Y, Yoshifuku S, Kihara T, Minagoe S, Tei C. (2002) Effect of repeated sauna therapy on survival in TO-2 cardiomyopathic hamsters with heart failure. *Am J Cardiol* 90:343-5.

[13] Ikeda Y, Biro S, Kamogawa Y, Yoshifuku S, Eto H, Orihara K, Yu B, Kihara T, Miyata M, Hamasaki S, Otsuji Y, Minagoe S, Tei C. (2005) Repeated sauna therapy increases arterial endothelial nitric oxide synthase expression and nitric oxide production in cardiomyopathic hamsters. *Circ J* 69: 722-9.

[14] Kihara T, Biro S, Imamura M, Yoshifuku S, Takasaki K, Ikeda Y, Otuji Y, Minagoe S, Toyama Y, Tei C. (2002) Repeated sauna treatment improves vascular endothelial and cardiac function in patients with chronic heart failure. *J Am Coll Cardiol* 39:754-9.

[15] Kihara T, Biro S, Ikeda Y, Fukudome T, Shinsato T, Masuda A, Miyata M, Hamasaki S, Otsuji Y, Minagoe S, Akiba S, Tei C. (2004) Effects of repeated sauna treatment on ventricular arrhythmias in patients with chronic heart failure. *Circ J* 68:1146-51.

[16] Kihara T, Miyata M, Fukudome T, Ikeda Y, Shinsato T, Kubozono T, Fujita S, Kuwahata S, Hamasaki S, Torii H, Lee S, Toda H, Tei C. (2009) Waon therapy improves the prognosis of patients with chronic heart failure. *J Cardiol.* 53(2):214-8.

[17] Kuwahata S, Miyata M, Fujita S, Kubozono T, Shinsato T, Ikeda Y, Hamasaki S, Kuwaki T, Tei C. (2011) Improvement of autonomic nervous activity by Waon therapy in patients with chronic heart failure. *J Cardiol.* 57:100-6.

[18] Miyata M, Kihara T, Kubozono T, Ikeda Y, Shinsato T, Izumi T, Matsuzaki M, Yamaguchi T, Kasanuki H, Daida H, Nagayama M, Nishigami K, Hirata K, Kihara K, Tei

C. (2008) Beneficial effects of Waon therapy on patients with chronic heart failure: results of a prospective multicenter study. *J Cardiol* 52:79-85.

[19] Node K, Kitakaze M, Yoshikawa H, Kosaka H, Hori M. (1997) Reduced plasma concentrations of nitrogen oxide in individuals with essential hypertension. *Hypertension* 30:405-8.

[20] Okada M, Hasebe N, Aizawa Y, Izawa K, Kawabe J, Kikuchi K. (2004) Thermal treatment attenuates neointimal thickening with enhanced expression of heat-shock protein 72 and suppression of oxidative stress. *Circulation* 109:1763-8

[21] Osada K, Imaizumi T. (2005) Heart Transplant Candidate Registry Committee of the Japanese Circulation Society. Special report from the heart transplant candidate registry committee in Japan. *J Heart Lung Transplant* 24: 810-4.

[22] Sasayama S, Asanoi H, Ishizaka S, Miyagi K. (1992) Evaluation of functional capacity of patients with congestive heart failure. In: Yasuda H, Kawaguchi H, editors. *New aspects in the treatment of failing heart.* Tokyo: Springer-Verlag; 113-7.

[23] Sillen MJ, Speksnijder CM, Eterman RM, Janssen PP, Wagers SS, Wouters EF, Uszko-Lencer NH, Spruit MA. (2009) Effects of neuromuscular electrical stimulation of muscles of ambulation in patients with chronic heart failure or COPD: a systematic review of the English-language literature. *Chest* 136:44-61.

[24] Takatani S, Matsuda H, Hanatani A, Nojiri C, Yamazaki K, Motomura T, Ohuchi K, Sakamoto T, Yamane T. (2005) Mechanical circulatory support devices (MCSD) in Japan: current status and future directions. *JArtif Organs* 8:13-27.

[25] Tei C, Horikiri Y, Park JC, Jeong JW, Chang KS, Tanaka N, Toyama Y. (1994) Effects of hot water bath or sauna on patients with congestive heart failure: acutehemodynamic improvement by thermal vasodilation. *J Cardiol.* 24 (3): 175-183. Japanese.

[26] Tei C, Horikiri Y, Park JC, Jeong JW, Chang KS, Toyama Y, Tanaka N. (1995) Acute hemodynamic improvement by thermal vasodilation in congestive heart failure. *Circulation.* 91(10):2582-2590.

[27] Tei C, Tanaka N. (1996) Thermal vasodilation as a treatment of congestive heart failure: a novel approach. *J Cardiol* 27:29-30.

[28] Tei C. (2007) Waon therapy: soothing warmth therapy. *J Cardiol* 49:301-4.

[29] Trotti R, Carratellegarbieri M, Micieli G, Bosone D, Rondanellego P. (2001) Oxidative stress and a thrombophilic condition in alcoholics without severe liver disease. *Haematologica* 86: 85-91.

[30] Weber AA, Silver MA. (2007) Heat therapy in the management of heart failure. Congest Heart Fail 13: 81-3

[31] Yoon SJ, Park JK, Oh S, Jeon DW, Yang JY, Hong SM, Kwak MS, Choi YS, Rim SJ, Youn HJ. (2011) A warm footbath improves coronary flow reserve in patients with mild-to-moderate coronary artery disease. *Echocardiography* 28:1119-24.